STANDING, SITTING, WALKING, RUNNING

Also by Jenny Beeken

YOGA OF THE HEART — A WHITE EAGLE BOOK OF YOGA
YOUR YOGA BODYMAP FOR VITALITY
YOUR YOGA BIRTHGUIDE
DON'T HOLD YOUR BREATH
ANCIENT WISDOM

ACKNOWLEDGMENTS

I would like to give acknowledgment and thanks to my editor and publisher, Colum Hayward, who has stood by me and encouraged me in the ideas for and the writing of this book, whatever I throw at him. I give great thanks to my teachers, Shri B. K. S. Iyengar, and then Vanda Scaravelli, through the wonderful classes of Diane Long and Sophy Hoare.

Also to Cittaviveka, Chithurst Buddhist Monastery, especially Ajahn Sucitto and Ajahn Karuniko for their brilliant Dhamma Talks; and again to the White Eagle Lodge, especially Joan Hodgson and Ylana Hayward.

I give my thanks to Patricia Lopez for her chapter on running and for staying with it all when it was much more than she had anticipated; to photographer Michael Prior and to those who came to be photographed: Patricia Lopez, Lisa Christensen, Will Lane and Thierry Lambert. I also give thanks to Jane Stockton, for the photographs from India

To Murray Nettle for her diligent, carefully considered, expressive drawings taken from her own thorough practice together with her artistic skills

For their written contributions: Ylva Wilding, Will Lane, Robert Barnes, Adam Brickley.

And to Winkie Harrison for her diligent, careful proof reading.

Standing, Sitting, Walking, Running

HOW YOUR POSTURE AFFECTS YOUR MIND

Jenny Beeken

with a chapter by Patricia Lopez
and drawings by Murray Nettle

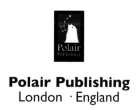

Polair Publishing
London · England

First published 2016
by Polair Publishing, London
www.polairpublishing.co.uk

British Library Cataloguing in Publication Data
A catalogue entry for this book is available from the British Library

ISBN 978-1-905398-33-1

Book Permissions
The publishers are grateful to Alistair Shearer and Rider and Co. for permission to use the excerpts on pp. 13 and 74 from his translation of THE YOGA SUTRAS OF PATANJALI; to Vedanta Press for the translation from the *Bhagavad Gita* by Swami Prabhananda and Christopher Isherwood on pp. 72-3; to Princeton Book Company, for the quotation from Mabel Elsworth Todd's book THE THINKING BODY, on pp. 39–40 ; to HealersLibrary.com and www. drbradleynelson.com for the quotation from Dr Bradley Nelson's THE EMOTION CODE on pp 69-70; to Pinter and Martin, for the excerpt on p. 19 from LIKE A FLOWER by Sandra Sabatini; to Amaravati Buddhist Monastery, Great Gaddesden, Herts, for permission to quote the excerpt from THE CHANTING BOOK on p. 76: as well as to the publishers and authors of the various short quotations

Set in Gill Sans by the publisher
and printed in Great Britain by
Halstan Publishing Group, Amersham

Contents

Introduction: Posture

We have within us the power to change our posture dramatically and this will transform our minds.

WALKING, standing, sitting and even running are everyday actions that we perform unconsciously, sometimes easily and sometimes in discomfort and pain. Either way, if we acted with awareness of what is involved in these movements – and the whole process is amazing when you feel it and study it – it would make an enormous difference to how we perform them, and to our bodies and how we feel. It would enable our posture to change. Our posture would improve by becoming more upright and our spines would find their natural length and curve. Then we can move from the spine, which is what nature intended: it is the backbone of the whole body – both literally and in the sense of 'the main support of a system'.

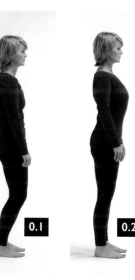

If our spine is not aligned and 'awake', we tend to move from the knee joint, which is then bearing too much weight down on it. The knee is not intended to bear weight – it is for movement, primarily.

If you look around at people's posture, especially if you see them on a mobile phone, as people so frequently are now, you can see how closed up and collapsed down their bodies have become. The pelvis sits too heavily down on the thighbones, creating strain on the knee joint; the ribs are too close to the pelvis, and the neck falls into the shoulders. The Western body is a sorry picture of our society, but it can change with some effort and mindfulness.

Ideally, this book would be superfluous, as it is about things we do 'naturally' and every day (even if our running is a quick sprint for a train or a bus!). How we do them is the interesting question, and why can all of them feel uncomfortable at times? Perhaps you will find some interesting questions and answers here; also, more aliveness and energy for these everyday issues!

If you practise yoga, and see it as a wholeness rather than a workout, it needs to address how we hold ourselves upright, and how we live with regard to our physical bodies, our minds, and our relation to other beings on our planet (and to the planet itself) in our daily lives.

'Holding ourselves upright' is a telling expression, indicating a tension required for us to remain in an upright position. Do other animals have to 'hold themselves' on four legs? Do fishes 'hold themselves' in the sea? What has happened to us that we need to 'hold ourselves upright'? Is it that it has become a strain, an effort, even to stand?

It is helpful to look first at the animal kingdom, and then at indigenous peoples that visibly stand, sit, and move with far less strain than we do. They do not seem to need to push, to expend effort like we do in Western civilization. Here, we have come to the point that we sit and stand in strain and discomfort, in a physical body that is collapsing (perhaps even in the same way as western civilization itself!).

Although you do not need to practise or study yoga in order to follow what is written here, this is a book about everyday awareness – or a mindfulness of how we live our everyday lives with respect to posture, breathing and attitude of mind. So it's essentially a book on the practice of yoga as a discipline within our daily life, and although some yoga poses are offered, it is mainly intended to encompass our day-to-day posture and how we move in largely natural activities such as walking, running, sitting, swimming, cycling and climbing, with contributions from people who engage in these activities regularly in their lives. In this respect, it is not so much a yoga book as one that uses the same

awareness of ourselves that yoga ideally offers.

The movements described are subtle, and generally very minimal, and can feel to be more about the direction behind them than actual movement – although there is still always some movement (for example, towards the earth, which has been described as 'the feet finding the earth underneath them'). In order to find the earth, the feet have to engage more with the ground as well as engage up through the ankle joint, the joint that connects the feet to the rest of the body. Yet these subtle movements are enormous in the effect that they can have on our minds, on our daily lives and our whole being. So do not be put off if at first you do not feel much happening in the movements described, and you find it difficult to connect to the body in this aware way. Do persevere, as these connections will come to you and eventually become natural.

They are *natural* because they are how the body would be without the *unnatural* things we do today. If you look at a body in a part of the world where people do not spend so much time in chairs and cars and hunched over computers, you will notice how aligned and upright the body tends to be. I remember looking at workers in India, poor people such as the one who swept all the paths where we were staying. As she worked she took her spine straight forward (just like the pose known in yoga as the triangle) and was very firm in the way her weight went down through her feet. As she was sweeping, it was clear that there was no strain in that body.

Another lady carried many branches of a tree on her

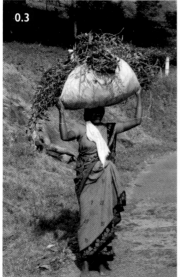

0.3

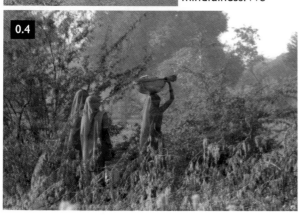

0.4

head, and with her aligned spine there was again no strain in her neck or head. The lumbar vertebrae and the legs and feet were giving support for her neck. The pictures (0.3, 0.4) show similar examples.

A way to get back to natural methods of using the body is to practise a spiritual discipline of meditation, awareness, mindfulness. We might choose the practice of the postures (*asanas*) of yoga, not as a workout but to address the ways in which our posture has become collapsed, weak, held and strained. Although these movements are subtle they will, to begin with, feel like hard work. This is because it takes tremendous focus to connect the mind to the body in this manner and then to engage bones, muscles, ligaments and tendons that are not used to working in such a way. But what we are seeking to access are all the natural movements that we have lost over time, so that it does become easier to connect to them and maintain them as time goes by. Patience and perseverance are needed, though! As we have tended to drag our bodies around by our heads and shoulders, by the same measure are we 'in our heads'.

Our posture is very affected by the attitudes we adopt in life as a result of the process of day-to-day living itself. For example, if we feel 'hard done by' and resentful we will be literally be 'down at heel' – that is, heavy on the feet, and on the knee and ankle joint. If we feel strong and victorious our chest and breastbone will be lifted and open. If we feel 'down at heart' that area will be literally closed in on itself, with the shoulders hunched in.

Attitudes are also expressed often very strongly in gestures that we make. We have ways of greeting one another, wishing good luck, waving good bye. A raised fist or two fingers up to the world tell us exactly the attitude behind the gesture. If they are negative, we do have the ability within us to change these attitudes, by first of all recognizing that that is what they are –

attitudes – rather than essentially *who* we are. Next, we can turn them around by taking more personal responsibility for how we feel, and how quickly this feeling can shift – by our going for a good walk, for example. I have used walking as a tool many times in writing this book, at times when I have felt stuck or unclear in my writing. Ideas and clarity in them come to me – very soon after starting out. The rhythm of the walk relaxes, clears and clarifies the mind.

The postures of yoga also change these attitudes naturally and gradually over time. For example, lifting the arms to open the armpits, allowing the lymph to move freely, has the effect of lifting the chest area out of the hips, so moving the spine and heart forward and up (0.5), thus changing a mood that might be one of depression. What we do with our hands and feet also can work on attitudes that are not serving us.

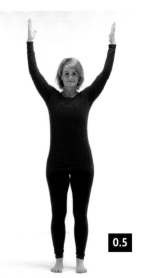

0.5

For instance, when walking you can maybe try to feel the pads of the toe tips connecting you up through your legs to your spine. This vital connection between the extremities of the body and its centre or core is used in yoga practice and meditation to focus us, so that we can become aware of the part of us that is conditioned by attitude. Such connections of the extremities of the body back to the centre in yoga are called 'mudras', which are an important concept in this book.

Mudras

I have mentioned how attitude affects our posture so that as we become more upright, more aligned in the spine, and more open across the shoulders and chest, so our attitude to life changes subtly, gradually, almost without us noticing at first. These are mudras of the body – *kaya* mudra – being demonstrated.

How we hold our hands is another form of mudra, *hasta* mudra, showing our attitude at the moment of doing it. Such mudras are part of our range of expressions towards one another. By using a particular position of the hand and fingers chosen to have

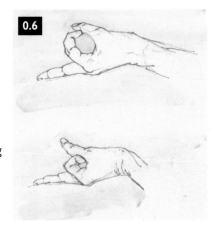

0.6

a specific effect on the whole body we can consciously change to how we really want to express ourselves.

There are even mudras of the feet – *pada* mudras. They are mudras of how we stand (or the way in which we place and connect to our feet to the earth underneath us). All these mudras can be deeply indicative of our selves.

To demonstrate such connections further, if you rub the tip of your thumbs over your fingertips, can you gradually feel a connection growing, back to your upper spine, and the chest and heart area? Touching thumb and fingertips connects the nerve endings in the body back to their source. What we do with one part of the body very much affects another, and thus the whole body. Both the fingertips and toetips connect us back to the spine – we take our awareness right out to our extremities and then back to our core.

The mudras of hand and feet and body connect back to and so affect the brain. For example *chin* mudra, which Patricia (Pachi) talks about in the context of running (p. 53), is where the tip of the index finger touches the tip of the thumb, very lightly (0.7, 0.8). This is like an electrical connection through the nervous system of the body, making a circuit up through the arms to the heart and head.

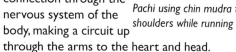

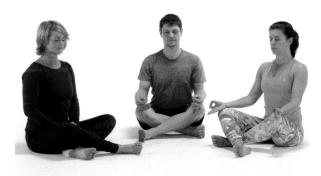

Pachi using chin mudra to relax the shoulders while running

Yoni mudra connects us to the earth and to the base of our spine. How amazing it is to find that runners of today are using this very ancient yoga practice to relax their shoulders and so run faster and easier from their legs, hips and feet!

In this book we will investigate how all the different mudras affect us and how we can employ and practice the specific mudras of yoga to change physical and mental attitudes that are not serving us. There will be plenty of mention of bones and muscles, too – accompanied by drawings that show where they are. If you want more detail, Wikipedia give excellent definitions and there are many good anatomy websites. One of the best books is THE ANATOMY OF MOVEMENT by

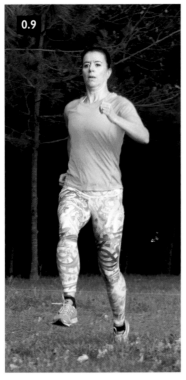

0.9

Blandine Calais-Germain.

For us to feel and understand how the body moves it does help to look at anatomy in terms of the bone structure and how the muscles connect and move over the bones. This way of moving, though, is different from the 'extend and contract' way that is generally employed. In yoga, we are asking the muscles to lengthen and 'engage' back to the bone. You only feel this with practice.

As an example, with the long thighbone and thigh muscles the description of one way of movement is 'to be aware that your thighs are getting thinner' as you 'engage' the muscles around and up the whole length of the thigh bone from the knee joint to the hip joint. In this way the back of the thighs, the group of hamstring muscles, are gathered in and up from below the knee joint right up to the buttock bones. At the front of the thighs, the strong quadriceps gather in and up from below the knees to the front of the pelvis. The inner thighs – the strong multiple adductor muscles – gather up towards the pubic bone and in towards the inner thighbone. The outer thigh – the iliotibial band – gathers in and up and back to the outer thighbone. In this way the whole thigh is being streamlined to stand more in and up into the hip joint, as Pachi shows in 0.9.

The muscles mentioned are described in more detail in the chapters, as they arise. Both mudras and breathing are addressed more fully in my book, DON'T HOLD YOUR BREATH (see reading list, p. 78).

Sitting

The later part of the final chapter, which is on 'Sitting', might also be headed 'meditation' and treated as a separate chapter. I have kept it as one chapter on 'sitting', as sitting is actually more challenging to the western body and mind than any movement! This is why – despite this book's title – the whole subject is treated last.

With the restlessness of our minds – especially apparent in the last twenty or thirty years, since we began to spend so much time on electrical devices, such as computers, mobile phones, playstations and televisions – the difficulty comes out particularly strongly when we sit with ourselves, with our minds that have been 'educated' to be so busy. Sitting with ourselves is an enormous undertaking for us, much more so than addressing our posture.

It is vital, at first, to address the posture of 'sitting', for if the spine is aligned (that is, the crown of the head is directly above the base of the spine), then the mind, which we consider to be in the brain, can relax and quieten. Sitting comes last because it is most helpful, even essential, to put into practice first what is said in the chapters on standing and walking; they will over time help align your sitting posture. For as soon as the body collapses and the alignment is lost, the mind goes off 'on a topic' into the future, into the past, which brings up anxiety, fear, worry, resentment – all of them natural human feelings which arise when we leave the present moment.

Sitting or meditation is about realizing that those worries are not the sum total of who we are. So the term, 'sitting' is used in many areas of practice and the first three chapters will be enormously helpful to 'Sitting' (chapter 4) and meditating. It is helpful to many people to consider they are 'sitting', especially if meditation feels to be impossible, although the intention to sit, whatever then happens, is itself meditation.

Yoga is the settling of the mind into silence.
When the mind has settled, we are established in our essential nature, which is unbounded consciousness.
Our essential nature is usually overshadowed by the activity of the mind.
THE YOGA SUTRAS OF PATANJALI, translated by Alistair Shearer

Chapter 1: Standing

The human spine is capable of growing in both directions just like a plant.
The lumbar area suffers most when standing incorrectly. The lumbar vertebrae
that become misaligned are crushed together by tension.
These compressed vertebrae pinch the nerves that pass through
the corresponding vertebral cavity, causing pain and muscular spasm.
We have to recreate the proper space between the vertebrae
so that the nerves can be released and health re-established.
AWAKENING THE SPINE (*Vanda Scaravelli*)

HAVE YOU noticed how quickly we develop the habit, as we grow older, of believing we have to grab onto handrails, push ourselves up from a chair using our hands and shoulders and lean on a support if our back is under strain, or feel strain in the knee joint when moving? This comes when we lose the awareness of how the downward movement of the feet, engaging them with the ground, gives the strength and 'standing up' of the legs.

It is the feet and legs, the

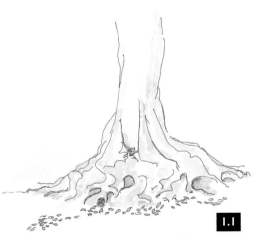

1.1

shinbone and thighbone connecting us to the spine, that are intended to support our weight. The knee joint is not primarily intended to be weight-bearing. Its main purpose is movement. We have tended to brace it back so that it becomes weight-bearing, for we have lost the connection to our feet – lost our sense of the arches of the feet, the ankle joint and the extrinsic muscles of the feet that connect them to our legs. We then have to pull ourselves up from the shoulders, neck and upper back – creating enormous unnecessary strain in those areas.

It is possible to change these habits, even if they are long term, with awareness and practice.

To gain the awareness let us ask ourselves this, first. In our standing posture, can we feel connection to the ground, the earth underneath us? Can we connect down through our feet and the base of our spine? The spine above the pelvis can then have the effect of taking the rest of the body up towards the heavens. It is just as Vanda Scaravelli states in the opening quotation. This is a gravitational balance within our bodies that requires 'engagement' rather than strain or even effort, at least in the way that we consider effort.

We have come to associate effort with pushing and straining. The derivation of the word 'effort', from Latin roots, offers *ex* which means out of or from, and *fortis*, which means strong or vigorous. Effort is what arises out of strength. It has the same meaning in Sanskrit, a language which stands behind Latin, much earlier in the sequence of the growth of language. Thus 'effort' is something which arises from being full of vigour, not from straining hard. A strong intention is needed to change and move the body, rather than an enforced and constrained 'effort' (using the word in the way so many people understand it). The postures of yoga, being firm and definite, have the power in them to wake up and move the body to a new way of standing – one that lifts us, giving a balance with gravity that is empowering and enlightening to the whole of ourselves.

However if we can stand, walk and sit, with

awareness and aliveness, connecting from our feet to the crown of our head, then that is enough: we do not need to do lots of postures unless we wish to, or if we practise a different discipline such as *tai chi* or *qi gong*, or gym training and aerobics.

Awareness

First of all, we need to be aware of our balance on our feet. It is helpful to have bare feet if possible as you discover this (you are likely to slip in socks, and shoes

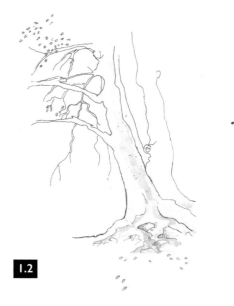

1.2

can restrict the movement of the toes) but it is still possible in both, as you might suddenly feel like bringing this awareness in when you are waiting in a queue or having to stand for some time. Are you heavy on your heels as you stand? Do you 'dig your heels in'? If so, can you come further forward onto the balls of your feet?

There are some very interesting expressions in the English language! Another is to be 'on the ball'. What does this mean? To be aware; alert, awake, ready for anything. Such expressions are extraordinarily literal, as coming forward more onto the ball of your foot really has that effect on the mind and on the awareness – on the whole self in fact. To balance the weight of the body between the ball of the foot and the heel is to be 'on the ball'.

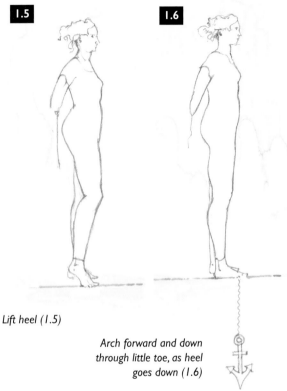

Lift heel (1.5)

Arch forward and down
through little toe, as heel
goes down (1.6)

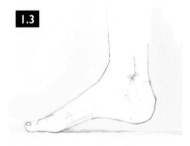

Heels slightly lifted so arch of foot is engaged,

then

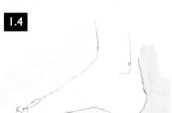

Arches retain their lift as heel comes very slightly forward and down

We can do this by lifting our heels slightly – just a millimetre or two (1.3). This allows the toes to spread forward and to feel the earth lightly, rather than 'gripping on for dear life'! Can you retain that movement of the heels as you bring them first gently forward and up and then down so engaging the arches of the feet (1.4)

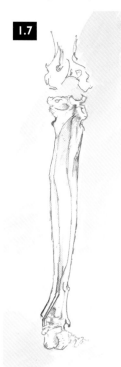

1.7

1.8

Medial view of tibialis posterior – to show attachment to footbones

Posterior view of tibialis posterior – a most important postural muscle – to show attachments to knee

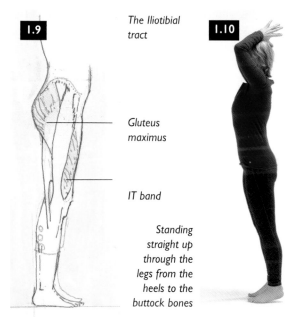

1.9

The *Iliotibial tract*

1.10

Gluteus maximus

IT band

Standing straight up through the legs from the heels to the buttock bones

to give you 'a spring in your step' – another of those useful expressions – as you walk? Now put your hands together and then your thumbs on the crown of your head, as Lisa is doing (1.10), and then come forward off your heels again, retaining the lift of the crown of the head into your thumbs as your heels come forward and down.

Now lift one heel, as shown (1.5), and feel the connection down into the little toe – your 'anchor' to the earth (1.6) – and then, as you take

the heel down feel the length back through the outside of the foot from the outer heel, and then up through the outer leg, via the deep *tibialis posterior* muscle (1.7, 1.8), from the foot to the knee and then along the outer thigh up into the hip joint.

Attached from the outer pelvis, along the thighbone, to below the outer knee joint with attachments there onto the length of the thighbone, is the iliotibial tract or band, often referred to as the 'IT band' (1.9).

It is made of strong fibrous fascia (see p. 24) which,

when connected and strengthened, enables the thigh to stand up into the hip joint so that the pelvis is free and acting as a shock absorber for the connection of the legs to the spine. (It also stabilizes the knee joint in walking and running.)

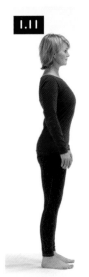

The *tibialis posterior* muscle and the IT band are among the most important components of the body posturally, as along with the other long thigh muscles they give the 'standing straight up' (1.11) position of the leg bones, rather than the braced-back position (1.12), of knee and calf muscle, which puts strain on the knee joint, calf muscles and the lower back and disconnects us to our feet.

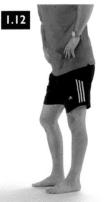

Then, from the *tibialis posterior* standing straight up, the hamstring group of muscles can also stand straight up from below the knee to the buttock bones, and through to the sacro-tuberous ligament that connects to the sacrum. This engages the strong bulky gluteus

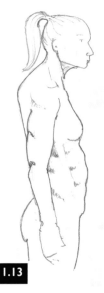

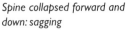

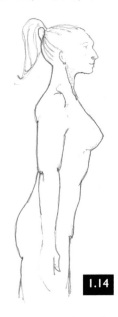

Spine collapsed forward and down: sagging

Spine engaging to the midline of the body: upright

(bottom) muscles to stand up and support the sacrum, so it is rested up and back. Once you have this, you will then never need a bottom lift! (The 'glutes' – the *gluteus maximus* muscles – tend to collapse in and down when the pelvis is collapsed).

You can now also see the difference that has come around the waist as well. In 1.13 the legs are not standing up to support the sacrum or the spine, while in 1.14 you can see the effect of standing up through the thigh bone, as well as engaging the buttock muscles. The deep spinal muscles engage back to the spine and this movement brings the more superficial abdominal muscles back to the spine and to the midline of the body.

What I have described is rather subtle and takes some time of focus and practice, but the posture does come with perseverance. It is also surprisingly hard work to just stand still and find inner movement that we have lost over years, so do not overdo it. Instead move, lie down, or do whatever your body feels it needs to do.

Standing with this specific awareness is termed *tadasana* in Sanskrit, which means 'as it is now' implying that 'as it is now' changes with each aware connection of the mind to the body and we can be present with this subtle change.

It is also called 'mountain pose' as we can feel we create a bridge between the earth underneath us and the heavens or the sky above us – just as a mountain can feel to be doing.

'Mountain pose is full of tiny and subtle shifts that rise up from the feet towards the head. It can be like a miniature earthquake that upsets any restrictive twist the body may have settled into. It is these postural weaknesses, twists and strange curves in the spine, and ways of standing and moving that have all imprinted themselves on the body, making the position difficult and tiring to maintain.

'For the first few months I found practising mountain pose very tiring, but then I moved into a state of greater calm and a deeper listening. Helped by Vanda's hands, I managed to bring my attention to the bottom of my feet and to breathe towards the soles and slowly develop a sense of roots…. I was beginning to get glimpses of the incredible intelligence that this active presence released. Maybe the origin of so much of my tightness and contraction, strains and pains was the lack of this continual attention.'

LIKE A FLOWER – MY YEARS OF YOGA WITH VANDA SCARAVELLI (Sandra Sabatini)

Lying Down

If standing causes you any strain at all – especially anywhere in your back or neck – then please lie down whenever you feel you need to, as this is hard work and we have a tendency to push our backs rather than engage our legs and feet. You can also start by lying down, or you can go to the instructions for sitting on a chair in chapter 4.

For lying down, use the floor if possible (if not, a firm bed) and have your feet against a wall (1.15). If this is uncomfortable on your back, bend your knees up to bring your feet flat on the floor as this keeps the feet active and connected to the legs and therefore the spine, and also helps overcome the tendency for one or both of the feet to flop out – which is caused by the hips being held tightly and unevenly. You thus create the same position as when you stand, except at ninety degrees. Put your hands behind your head to lift it, and look to check whether your knees are pointing up towards the sky or ceiling, so that they are aligned with the hips. Also, ease your neck out with your hands as you bring your head back down.

Now feel the position of the ankle joint, the hip joint, the shoulder joint, and then the ears: are they all in line? This is how we need to be when standing; if your back is under strain you are likely to have the top of the pelvis too far forward so that the lumbar spine collapses forward and down onto the sacrum.

There is a tendency then to try and flatten the lumbar back towards the floor. This is very hard work and an unnatural position for the lumbar spine, as there should be a curve in it, but a curve that is lengthened

up more and back to the midline of the body (1.14).

If you will now spread the feet into the wall (or ground if your knees are bent) feel how that engages the thighbone up into the hip joint, which then takes the tailbone (the coccyx) down towards your heels and lifts the lumbar region up off the sacrum towards the crown of the head. This two-way movement of the spine is vital to standing, walking, running and sitting. Do you feel the spine spread and relax the upper back down and ease the neck out of the shoulders? Relax there, feeling the sacrum bone and back of the skull (the occipital bone) resting back into the ground without you having to push anywhere or 'do it' in a way that comes from the will.

Feel now how you are breathing, exploring whether the diaphragm can spread and open as you inhale and relax and soften as you exhale. Feel the back ribs spread

1.15

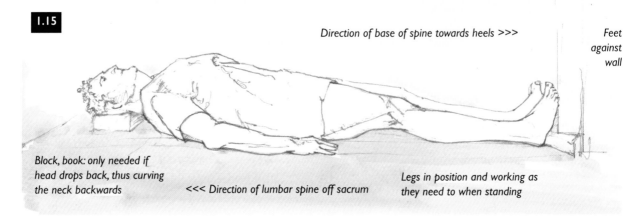

Direction of base of spine towards heels >>>

Feet against wall

Block, book: only needed if head drops back, thus curving the neck backwards

<<< *Direction of lumbar spine off sacrum*

Legs in position and working as they need to when standing

away from the spine on the floor as you inhale and rest as you exhale. Relax here and focus on your breathing for a while to feel how it is moving through your body, without forcing it at all.

When you are ready to get up, roll onto your side, put a support in the form of your arm or cushion under your head, adjust there for a moment or two, and then come to sitting for another moment or two. Then you could do the chair movements (pp. 58-61) or return to standing, recreating the awareness and position of the hips, shoulders and spine from when you were lying down.

Using the Wall

Another way to find alignment and relieve any strain is to stand, but rest into a wall with the knees bent so that the back is gently rested but not pushed into the wall. Do not push the head back either, but see where it naturally sits. Rest your palms flat back on the wall – resting, feel your breath there for a moment or two. Do your upper back and head rest back or curl forwards off the wall? If you spread your feet into the ground and hands into the wall, your spine then comes forward and up, lifting the top of your breastbone towards your head (1.16). This may have the effect of bringing your hips naturally and easily off the wall so that your upper back and head then rest back into it. It's important that you don't *push* the hips off the wall: rather, let the movement of the spine forward relax the shoulders out

and down and so ease the neck out of the shoulders. Relax there, feeling the sacrum bone and back of the skull (the occipital bone) resting back into the ground without you having to push anywhere or 'do it' in a way that comes from the will (1.17).

Feel now how you are breathing, exploring whether the diaphragm can spread and open as you inhale and relax and soften as you exhale. Feel the back ribs

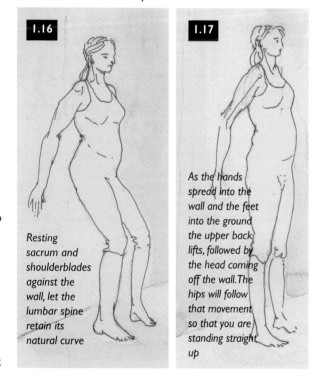

1.16

Resting sacrum and shoulderblades against the wall, let the lumbar spine retain its natural curve

1.17

As the hands spread into the wall and the feet into the ground the upper back lifts, followed by the head coming off the wall. The hips will follow that movement so that you are standing straight up

spread away from the spine as you inhale and relax back as you exhale.

Then rest the hips back onto the wall again, keeping the awareness of the spine lifting forward and up under the breastbone to the top towards the crown of the head. Has the upper back and head stayed more rested back onto the wall?

Can you feel how we tend to push the lower back ribs in so that the front lower ribs and bottom of the breastbone (the *xiphisternum*) then push forward and the top of the breastbone collapses in? We need to reverse that. Resting back into the back ribs will allow the kidneys and the adrenal glands (which sit on the top of the kidneys) to relax back more and so rest us back into the back of the body. We tend to be pushed into the front part of the body, especially in the pelvis, abdominal area and lower ribs and chin. If we were more rested back and broad in the back area we would not be under the same strain in our bodies or minds and actually more efficient, as we would not feel so rushed in all we do. The American expression 'laid back' expresses this literally and although it means 'relaxed', we can relax more easily if the physical body is more spread and open at the back rather than pushed forward towards the front.

In order to keep going and doing – achieving, rushing around through our day – we tend to have the adrenal glands, which sit just above the kidneys, on overcharge. This is actually a way of exhausting ourselves. I was amazed when I looked at my mother's medical notes just before she died, to discover that she had chronic kidney disease. When I asked the district nurse about this, she said quietly that all old people have chronic kidney disease! Is this, I wonder, because we put ourselves under such strain and push forward in this area?

Now spread down through your feet and up through your crown, spreading your hands firmly into the wall to lift yourself off the wall 'all in one piece' so that you still feel that spread into the back of the body when you return to standing. Now return to the instructions on standing and walking without strain but do not overdo anything. Rest, lying down or sitting, whenever you feel the need.

The Two-way Movement of the Spine or Vertebral Column

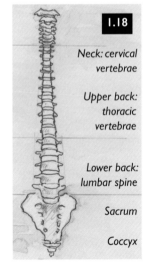

1.18

Neck: cervical vertebrae

Upper back: thoracic vertebrae

Lower back: lumbar spine

Sacrum

Coccyx

'Vertebral column' is an appropriate term for the spine, as it is a stack of vertebrae, thirty-three in all, from the base of the column right up to the head.

As I mentioned in the section on lying down, and as Vanda Scaravelli indicated in the quote at the beginning of this chapter, there is a two-way movement in this column. The first way (as shown by the downward arrow in 1.20) is down through the base of the spine, with gravity, from the bottom of the sacrum, with the firm downward movement of the feet, especially the heels. This in turn gives a second movement (as shown in upward arrow in the same drawing): a release of the big lumbar vertebrae off the top of the sacrum, which continues up into the upper back and neck. The strong standing up of the thigh bone into the hip joint helps create this movement all the way along the spine.

As a result of this two-way movement, the lumbar curve comes back to the midline of the body. The neck responds to this movement by easing up into its lesser curve, to bring the head up and back. It then sits it down on the broad atlas vertebra (1.19).

This is vitally important. Can you feel how the massive lumbar vertebrae (in comparison to the narrow cervical or neck vertebrae) actually have the job of holding the upper body and head up?

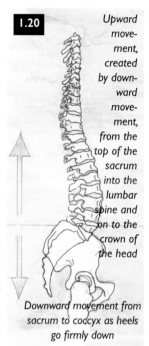

1.20

Upward movement, created by downward movement, from the top of the sacrum into the lumbar spine and on to the crown of the head

Downward movement from sacrum to coccyx as heels go firmly down

The two-way movement of the lumbar spine

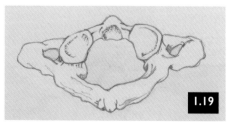

Atlas vertebra, which the head rests on

1.19

This is why the legs and feet need to be alive and connected through the pelvis to the lumbar vertebrae. The body below the diaphragm supports and lifts the body above the diaphragm so that it is free to move through the very mobile shoulder girdle.

We have got into a habit of holding ourselves up from our head, neck and shoulders, which is very hard work and causes all sorts of strain, as well as problems like frozen shoulder, arthritis in the neck vertebrae and tightness in the jaw, for it is not what nature intended the upper body to be doing. The upper body is for freedom and expression of movement – hugging, kissing, gestures, eating, speaking – not holding you up! It is not however helpful to try and move this area at the outset. Leave it alone to begin with, and address the posture of the lower body, as otherwise we will tend to move from the neck and shoulders to get there fast and 'do it'. This will make us push the spine at the lumbar and neck vertebrae and cause strain and pain.

After a good period of practice the habit will develop of standing down through the feet. This brings the thighbones standing up into the hip joint and connects to the spine, bringing it forward and up through the relaxed shoulders to stand the head upright. Then the spine moves through the relaxed shoulders to stand the head upright. When the spine stands up into its rightful position the upper body can then relax out of its strain and move in a freeing, softening way.

Muscles that Support the Standing up of the Spine

Back to the feet: now feel the spread across the ball of the foot from the little toe joint to the big toe joint and the connection back to the inner heel and up the inner leg to the multiple adductor muscles (1.26) on the inner thighs – so that you are taking the inner thighs up and out away from one another, lifting and spreading up to the pubic bone. This again opens and releases the whole pelvis up off the head of the femur (thighbone).

So now, with this inner, outer and back-of-the-leg connection, we can begin to feel the connection of the feet and legs to the spine. It is as though the pelvis can now float and relax in the fascia. Fascia is defined as 'a sheet of connective tissue covering or binding body structures such as muscles'. It is often likened to 'cling film' in its role of holding together the structure of the body. And so we go through the pelvis to the spine, engaging from the deep *psoas* muscle, which connects from the top inner thigh all the way up each lumbar vertebra

*Psoas
(connects leg
to lumbar
spine)*

1.21

Multifidus

Front (anterior) view   Back (posterior) view

to the diaphragm and the twelfth thoracic vertebra.

This awareness has the effect of engaging the deep spinal muscles – the *multifidus* (which interestingly are the most powerful muscles in the body, 1.21, 1.22) – to bring the strength back into the large lumbar vertebrae, so it stands upright in its natural curve but much more back to the midline of the body. Otherwise it is pushed forward into a lordosis or flattened back in an attempt to relieve strain there. These deep core muscles then naturally engage the muscles that are nearer the surface, such as the *rectus abdominis* (1.24), the oblique and transverse and *quadratus lumborum* (1.25) so that we have our own natural corset holding us up, rather than a contracted six-pack (1.23). Now lift slightly off the

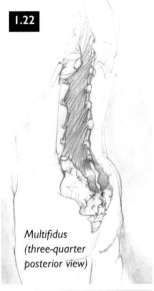

1.22

*Multifidus
(three-quarter
posterior view)*

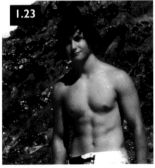

1.23

Contracted six-pack collapses spine forward and hunches upper back

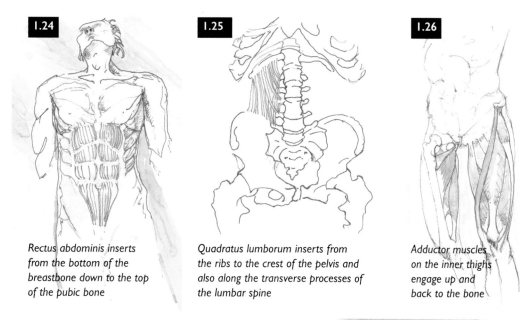

Rectus abdominis inserts from the bottom of the breastbone down to the top of the pubic bone

Quadratus lumborum inserts from the ribs to the crest of the pelvis and also along the transverse processes of the lumbar spine

Adductor muscles on the inner thighs engage up and back to the bone

the base of the spine is in line with the crown of the head.

As you lift the heels again, feel the connection all the way up the outside of the body from the little toe joint to the outer thigh, right up to the side ribs, so that maybe the arms feel they want to move up and out. But they are lifting from underneath, not being dragged up from the tightening of the muscles across the tops of the shoulders. This

heels again (a millimetre or two is enough), and feel how the whole upper body above the diaphragm lifts up off the pelvis and lumbar spine. Keep that lift as the heels come gently but firmly forward and down. Can you feel the connection and release that comes to the upper spine and breastbone?

Lift the heels again and feel how the upright breastbone and upper back bring the head up and back and then sit it lightly down on the top of the neck vertebrae, so that the head is lightly held up by the whole spine – particularly the strong lumbar spine – and

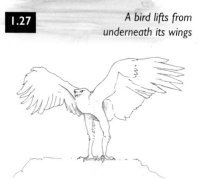

A bird lifts from underneath its wings

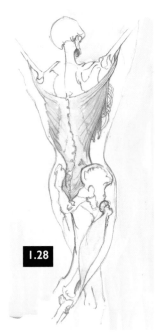

1.28

We too have a wing-like muscle, the latissimus dorsi, that lifts the arms from underneath (1.28, 29)

out and maybe up from this muscle, like a bird taking off?

Only lift your arms as high as you can do without straining. If you move as described, from the feet all

is very important, as so many people have strain across the shoulders and neck, and such conditions as frozen shoulders are caused by lifting just from the upper body rather than from the whole body. We have a wonderful wing-like muscle that has its origin just under the arms and connects down via strong fascia to the base of the spine. It is the latissimus dorsi.

Can we move the arms

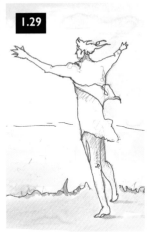

1.29

the way up the body, then the movement will gradually become easier and more natural, relieving shoulder and neck strain, but it is important not to overdo any of this at first as habits can be hard to break.

This movement, which opens up the armpits, can have a dramatic effect on our state of mind. When we feel under strain – held together, 'down', depressed – then we hold our arms tight into our chests. This hunches the upper back and restricts the flow of lymph (the lymph nodes are in the armpits) so then our energy gets stuck and restricted. When you open your arms your energy shifts, lightening your mood, freeing your heart.

Try this movement out on the dew drenched grass early in the morning. It has the power to transform your day!

Breathing

Are you ever aware of your breathing?

How do you breathe? Do you notice any strain as you do so? Do you notice if you hold your breath or if you do not breathe in or out fully?

How our breath moves through our body is affected directly by our posture as we will see and feel. The way we breathe exactly reflects what is happening in our body, our mind, our feeling senses, and our awareness of the world around us.

You may have noticed how the instructions given for standing from the feet upwards into the spine have

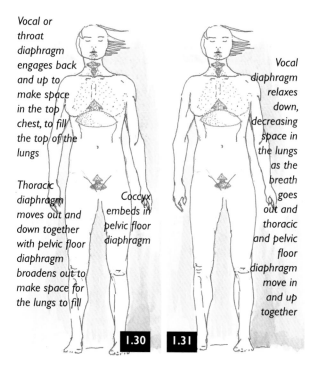

Vocal or throat diaphragm engages back and up to make space in the top chest, to fill the top of the lungs

Thoracic diaphragm moves out and down together with pelvic floor diaphragm broadens out to make space for the lungs to fill

Coccyx embeds in pelvic floor diaphragm

1.30

Vocal diaphragm relaxes down, decreasing space in the lungs as the breath goes out and thoracic and pelvic floor diaphragm move in and up together

1.31

Inhalation (breathing in)   *Exhalation (breathing out)*

opened out the rib cage, so that you can now breathe more easily. Can you now feel that the movement of the *latissimus dorsi* muscle (the one that is like wings) up from the coccyx to under the armpits tends to bring the breath in? If so, the breath, rather than being pulled in from the nostrils and top chest, will come more from the diaphragms of the body – which is what

nature intended. The diaphragms are very strong tendinous muscles. One of their 'jobs' is to keep the organs of the body in place – so, for example, the thoracic diaphragm stops the lungs and heart from falling into the abdomen! Their other role is in breathing. See drawings 1.30-32 for their position and names.

Because our western bodies tend to be collapsed down on the thighs and pelvis, we have difficulty breathing in a natural way, and so we pull the breath in from the abdominal area and/or the upper chest, shoulder and neck muscles (such as the pectorals and deltoids, intended to be used at the top of the breath and known as the secondary respiratory muscles). This has been likened to 'digging the garden with a kitchen fork' (a phrase from THE ART OF BREATHING by Donna Farhi)! See the drawing overleaf (1.33).

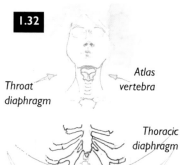

1.32

Throat diaphragm

Atlas vertebra

Thoracic diaphragm

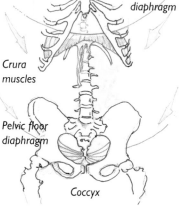

Crura muscles

Pelvic floor diaphragm

Coccyx

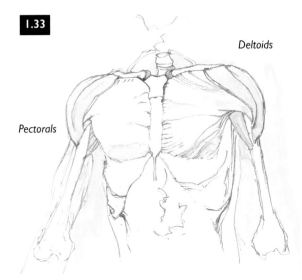

1.33

Deltoids

Pectorals

Overdeveloped secondary respiratory muscles that pull the breath in from the top of the chest

When our posture changes, then our breathing changes. We will breathe with the primary respiratory muscles, which are the diaphragms of the body, together with the intercostal muscles. Many other muscles around the abdomen are also involved in breathing, especially the *crura* muscles.

The thoracic diaphragm is likened to a parachute that is held down along the length of the lumbar spine to the sacrum by the long crura muscles. So as the *psoas* muscle engages back to the spine, the *crura* muscles engage and open the diaphragm out to create space

in the area above the diaphragm (1.32). This creates a vacuum in the lungs so the breath has to come in. There are several ways that the impulse to breathe in is created: one is the level of carbon dioxide in the blood, but another is a vacuum created in the lungs. Also, the pelvic floor diaphragm has to move with the thoracic diaphragm to instigate the inhalation and exhalation.

You can see in the drawing on the previous page (1.32) how the coccyx is embedded in the pelvic floor, so that as the coccyx and the heels root down towards the ground, the pelvic floor spreads and the *psoas* muscle engages up the sides of the lumbar spine, lengthening it. This has the effect of engaging and lengthening the *crura* muscles down, parachuting the thoracic diaphragm out, taking the ribs out with it, and making space for the lungs to open and fill with the breath.

At the same time, the neck vertebrae respond to the lengthening of the lumbar vertebrae, and the skirt-like *scalene* muscles around the neck engage and bring the neck to its natural curve, so that the vocal diaphragm in the throat domes up,

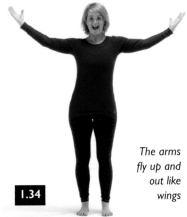

1.34

The arms fly up and out like wings

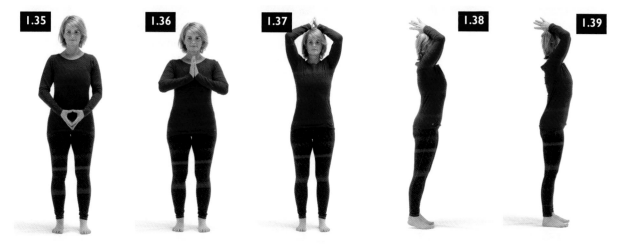

giving more space for the top of the chest then to fill.

If we let the movement come from the feet through the whole body, then the diaphragm will open and the breath will have space to come naturally in and out. The *latissimus dorsi* muscle will make the arms feel as though they want to fly up and out (1.34), but only go as far as you can without strain or tightening, or pulling from the secondary respiratory muscles. It doesn't matter how far this movement goes, and if you do it regularly then the strained shoulder joint and top muscles will gradually be able to relax, as they become more permanently supported from underneath, so strain and tension will go. This takes time and awareness in a practice and in everyday life.

You can pause, breathe out, and consciously let the shoulders broaden out to the side, so that the breastbone can lift and open. Then, as the diaphragm is very open in this position, the breath will easily come in again and maybe the arms will respond and move more as you exhale. But let it happen from the feet rather than pulling up from the shoulders. As you exhale, keep the lift and openness of the breastbone, so that the shoulders relax but stay broad and opened out to the side rather than down, as then they will not pull the upper thoracic spine forward and down.

Then come through the centre of the body, bringing the fingertips together in *yoni* mudra (1.35, 1.40)

Feel the movement that this mudra gives, which is of the feet spreading down into the earth with gravity. It then gives the standing up through the thighbones that make the hands want to travel up through the front of the body to *namaste* hands over the breastbone (1.36) with the upward lengthening of the spine.

As the hands reach the breastbone, feel the lift of the top of the breastbone into the little fingers. Can you feel this come through from the lumbar spine, engaging back to the midline of the body?

Feel how easily the diaphragm can open in this position, so that the breath has space to come in. Then when the arms want to move again, bring the little fingers onto the crown of the head (1.37).

Lift off the heels again, and once more feel this has the effect of bringing the head up and back and sitting it down on the top of the neck vertebrae (1.38). Keep that lengthening as the heels come down, and as the tailbone (coccyx) goes down with the heels but the crown of the head stays moving up into the little fingers (1.39). Feel how much the legs and lumbar vertebrae need to engage to retain this alignment and connection of the base and the crown. Then rest and relax the arms out and down.

The two movements, one of spreading the arms to the side and the other of bringing the fingertips together and coming in and up through the centre, are known jointly as 'The Tree of Light' or 'Tree of Life'

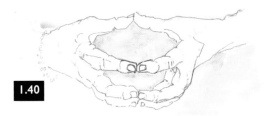

1.40

breath. This gives a complete movement out and then through the centre of the body. It is often practised by lifting from the shoulders, so that the naming is given at the end, as it is much more a movement through the whole body if it is practised in stages as described.

As you practise this, you may gradually become aware of the connection from the limbs to the spine, and even from the extremities of the body – the toetips and fingertips. Can you connect them back through the limbs and joints to the centre of the body, to the spine?

We can feel dragged down and out through the limbs – but there is a movement out and then a connection back in again. This is like life: we go out to the world around us, but then we need to connect back in again to ourselves. It is also the practice in sitting (see chapter 4, on sitting).

Take a moment or two now to feel how you are standing. What effects have the movements had on your posture? Is there a change in the way you are now? Is there any awareness of how you are breathing? And any sense that that has changed at all?

In Sanskrit, as we saw, standing like this is called *tadasana*, 'as it is now'. So how is it now on all levels of mind, body and consciousness? One of the reasons it is known as mountain pose is that a mountain stands firm, serene and upright.

Next become aware again of how you are breathing. Do you find that your breath comes in more naturally as your posture changes? We tend to want to do breathing exercises or try to breathe as we feel we should, but there is no way we can find our natural rhythm of the

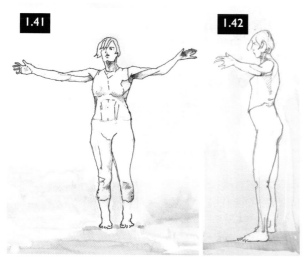

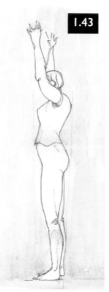

The arms might go up as the spine comes forward and up

the putting one foot in front of the other (an amazing action when you understand how it is achieved) takes us along, with the earth seeming to come up to meet the downward force of gravity as we move over the earth.

However, every one of the instructions and practice of awareness given can be taken into all of life's activities, be they considered work or play – from housework to gardening or swimming to sailing, or from football to tennis, or mountain climbing to surfing. At the end of a three-day yoga course I

breath by trying to impose a new pattern of breathing on an already strained one. However, if our posture changes so that the diaphragms move as we breathe, then we naturally and more easily breathe with our natural rhythm. We only need to be aware of this rather than try to change it, for it can cause all sorts of strain in the body if we 'try' to breathe.

You are now ready to walk with your new posture, which is less hard work than all the concentration and effort we have just put into standing still. The rhythm of

taught for IBM staff, one man said it gave him a state of consciousness similar to what sailing gave him. There used to be two players in the doubles tournament at Wimbledon that would sit upright and meditate for a minute or two between rounds of tennis. Then there is dancing in its myriad forms, which too can bring a meditational awareness alongside a body-based one.

On another hill we had pointed out to us the images of men dancing to a shaman playing his pipes. I was drawn to this figure. I thought of our own dancing days in those tiny sweaty cells in Lebanon. Like that shaman on the hill, I too believe that dancing is divine. It is the great liberator.
Brian Keenan, remembering being a hostage in the Lebanon, in BETWEEN EXTREMES (with John McCarthy)

Other activities

Cycling and Yoga by Will Lane...

I am a forty-four-year old yoga teacher and gardener, and father to a seven-year-old daughter, Bella. My interest in yoga and martial arts developed during my twenties, when I spent eight years in and around South East Asia, mainly Thailand. For my personal wellbeing, in addition to my daily yoga and meditation practice, I find great release comes from a few hours out on my bike to see the countryside, to breathe fresh air and to challenge myself – be it in a road race or climbing a tough hill. It is a powerful way to shift energy and clear the mind and subsequently relax deeply.

Cycling potentially involves extended periods of time sitting in one position, which can lead to tight quads, hamstrings and lower back, as well as to the shoulders rounding in and restricted movement in the spine.

So what can we do and how could we bring our awareness from yoga to the way we ride?

First, the bike set-up needs to be addressed. The saddle needs to be at the correct height so the pelvis is stable and not rocking. The fore/aft (forward/backward) movement of the saddle has to be adjusted correctly in order to keep the hip flexors open. The frame size and stem need to be the correct size/length which will avoid overreaching for the handlebars and a closing in of the chest and shoulders. A quality bike shop will offer a 'bike fit' service. There are various systems and I recommend this fit for any serious rider.

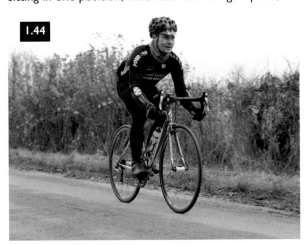

1.44

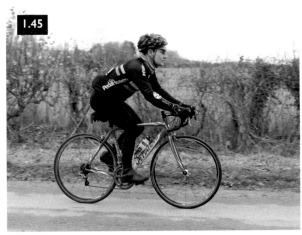

1.45

That's the bike part, then, so what can we do with our bodies to help?

If you are a regular practitioner of yoga and used to supporting yourself – that is, always being lifted in a posture in the ways Jenny describes – you will have begun to develop strength in your spine and gained awareness of the natural curves and shape of the spine. This shape is maintained when seated in cycling. From the hips, the sacrum tilts forward and the spine follows (quite straight) from sacrum to neck. The hands grip the bars lightly with the elbows bent and the shoulderblades down, released, while the chest and collar bones should remain open. Note that when the upper spine is lifted the back of the neck remains lengthened and hence is much softer.

...and by Robert Barnes

The ability to travel under one's own energy and in a way that connects to the elements for me is fundamental in cultivating a free spirit. I always feel young at heart when riding a bike, and love the feeling of the wind blowing through my hair. Often I will take to the bike as a form of therapy, through which I can alter my mood.

The energy created through yoga practice can be transferred directly onto the bike. The seated position adopted can be viewed as a yoga posture, and the breathing that occurs during riding can be viewed as energy cultivation. The feeling of freedom and connection with one's environment is like a meditation. The feeling of the propulsion of the bike comes through

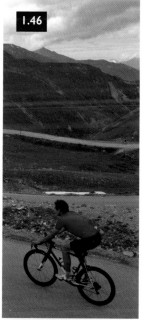

1.46

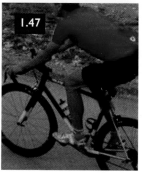

1.47

the elasticity of the spine and with the energy from the pelvis through the legs.

In cycling there is a tendency for the calf muscles to develop and to tighten. The lengthening down of the heels in yoga, and specifically the ability of the Achilles tendon to extend and maintain elasticity will prevent tight calves while cycling (1.47).

So notice when riding if the heels are lifting. This may happen more so if cycling shoes are used. Riding with lifted heels is a bit like walking in high heels. For the heels to drop the arches of the feet need to be lifted, but critically the Achilles tendon needs to let go, away from the heelbone, and not to tighten right through to the calf muscles. So keep the heel down. The angle of the foot will then determine the alignment of the knees and hips during the pedalling motion.

In general the foot becomes more active through the practices given in this book and/or through a good yoga practice. The arches of the feet and the ankle will be able to hold themselves up, and then when riding the leg motion right from the foot will free up the hips.

Yoga in the Water by Ylva Wilding

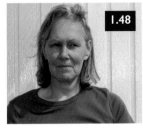

For me, yoga has brought alleviation from depression and arthritis, but much more than that it has brought a deeper connection between body and mind (and spirit) and has been a process of improving my own relationship with myself – by discouraging negative patterns of thinking and behaviour. Also it has brought the recognition that the body has its own wisdom and the learning to honour that wisdom. Here are some observations while floating in the Turkish Mediterranean.

Stretching out along one leg and spreading into the sole of the foot while allowing the other leg to relax bending the knee upwards … then changing sides. Spreading into the other foot and bending up the other knee … continuing to alternate between left and right sides … gradually bending knee more and bringing foot higher up leg. Towards the knee … then the groin…. As this movement begins there is a gentle swaying motion from side to side; as it is exaggerated so the swaying becomes a rotation. As this happens, there is a wonderful freedom of movement through the entire length of the spine … from the pelvis through the legs along to the feet … and from the shoulders along the arms to the hands….

D. H. Lawrence wrote, '*Look he hath movement upward! He spirals!*' (GOD IS BORN).

My experience reminded me of 'a rotary movement of atoms or particles of subtle matter round an axis, or the matter itself in rotation, such phenomena accounting for the formation of the universe and the relative motion of its parts.' (Descartes).

Climbing by Adam Brickley

In my experience, the biggest factor affecting confidence in climbing is perceived ability against perceived risk. Perceived ability can have an effect on actual ability, and a climber who wrongly perceives a route to be right on their limit, may grip harder through fear. This causes more energy to be expended, resulting in early fatigue.

Risk, in general, is very personal. I tend to feel that perceived risk and perceived ability tend to feed back into each other. A negative appraisal of your own ability will make the climb seem more dangerous than it is, and by definition more risky.

An overly conservative appraisal of the risk can cause more fear: hanging about on routes, getting tired, losing confidence and generally lowering your climbing ability. Needless to say, this is just scratching the surface,

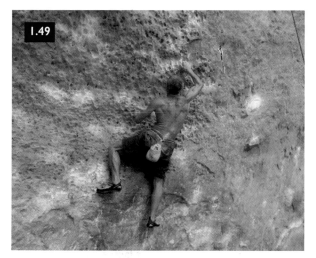

1.49

However, although climbers need to have a good range of movement, the real benefit of a yoga or posture-aware practice to the physical aspect of climbing is in getting the body to work and extend.

Typically during mindfulness practice we focus on the quality of the breath. Focusing on an extended outbreath can engage the parasympathetic nervous system. Having practised at home in a safe situation we can use this skill to encourage a return to calm in the emotions in a series of moves between bolts or gear placement.

In my view, developing a mindful awareness of movement can be equally beneficial to climbers. This can be developed by specific mindfully based bodywork such as yoga, or by intentionally trying to develop this while training against the wall. Every training session is an opportunity to practise dynamic body mindfulness, and can have practical applications in climbing – for example, placing attention on how the shifting centre of gravity affects the force required to stay on a hold, or trying climbing without hands on less steep sections.

Put your attention into becoming very aware of the feeling when in your body while making moves at your grade limit. Becoming very aware of how this feels can give you added confidence outside and maybe a way to avoid over-gripping, which leads to fatigue. Training dynos, in the climbing gym, where the climber leaves the wall completely to catch a hold out of reach, can be practised inside, with the benefits of a safe landing, until you are totally familiar with the feeling of taking off, the feeling in the air and making contact with the rock and catching a hold.

but it should seem obvious that the state of mind and emotional state are major factors in comfortable climbing at your realistic grade, and training the mind and emotions could be a valuable addition to a training programme.

Mindfulness meditation and bodywork do just this. Mindfulness meditation involves applying attention to present-moment stimuli while maintaining a non-judgmental attitude. During mindfulness meditation the meditator assumes a static posture to suit their body type, whereas bodywork is more dynamic. The dynamic forms may include many forms of yoga, Feldenkrais, Alexander technique, *tai chi* or a mindful attitude to any training programme; this list is certainly not exhaustive.

Yoga and climbing can complement each other.

Chapter 2: Walking

I only went out for a walk, and finally concluded to stay out till sundown, for going out, I found, was really going in.

John Muir

I began by heading west, out along the pointing arm of the Lleyn Peninsula of North Wales, to a remote island where the first glimmerings of a wild consciousness could be found.

THE WILD PLACES (Robert Macfarlane)

WALKING is one of the most wonderful actions of our human bodies, indeed of any body among the mammals of the planet, for as you walk you can feel just what is happening to the body and the effect it has on the mind and the whole self. Why do we feel 'impelled' to go out a for a walk when the mind is in a quandary or feeling stuck, stuffed up? Because the rhythm of the walk, the effect it has on the spine and the stimulation it gives to the cerebral spinal fluid has a clearing, balancing, 'sorting out' effect on the mind. So if we are upset or disturbed in any way the rhythm will balance that out, not suppressing it at all but processing it through our whole body, mind and emotions so that we can then act on the quandary or upset appropriately (and not from the kneejerk reaction).

It has been discovered recently that the instigation of the movement of the cerebral spinal fluid up the spine and into the brain comes from the sacrum bone, which moves in a rhythm from left to right as we step from one foot to the other, and so sends a pulse through the fluid to start its journey up the spine.

As well as on the mind, walking will of course have an enormous effect on the whole body: more or less every bone, muscle and ligament of the body will be employed (especially if you follow the directions of this chapter!), and in the process the digestive system, the respiratory system, the reproductive system, the circulatory system and the nervous system will all be toned, stimulated and balanced.

We now 'go out for a walk' if we 'find the time' to do so, whereas a hundred years ago we would have walked miles to post a letter or visit a friend. For example, you can read in Dorothy Wordsworth's journals, how she and her brother, the poet William Wordsworth, would walk twice daily from Grasmere to Ambleside to pick up their post, a round trip of nearly seven miles, and in addition take detours around the lakes to visit friends! How many of us do that sort of thing today?

Movements involved in Walking

From your new standing pose, take a single step: your own, comfortable walking step forward (2.1). Pause, and feel how the back heel turns in slightly. Now come more onto the outside of both feet, so that you feel the whole of the outside of the foot, from the little toe to the outer heel, firm on the ground. Can you feel how this takes the inner thighs up and away from one another?

Keep that movement up and out as you spread from the little toe joint to the big toe joint of both feet, letting the toes rest and feel the earth, rather than grip it. Feel the 'standing straight up' of the legs into the hip joint, the sensation that this gives. Now lift up through

the back heel as though you are going to take another step forward. Feel the lift of the thighbone into the hip joint more strongly and keep the same standing up and out of the thighbone as the heel goes back down. Lift up through the heel of the front foot, again feeling the lift that gives of the thighbone into the hip joint and maybe the arms want to fly up and out from underneath too? (2.2, 2.3)

Keep that lift as the heel goes down. How much has this affected your spine and your upper back? Have they moved more forward and up, so that your shoulders then relax out and away from the collarbone?

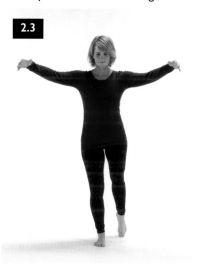

Then lift both heels together, keeping all the life, lift and standing up of the long thighbone which

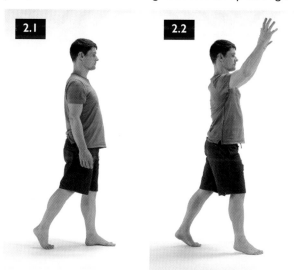

that gives you through the whole body as your heels come lightly forward and down.

Lift the back heel again and feel how that propels you forward now from the legs, to bring the back leg forward. Repeat on the other side.

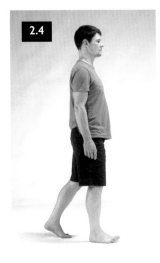

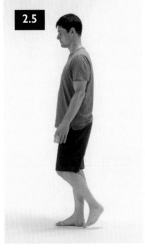

Shoulders broadening and relaxing out

Shoulders pulling spine down

You will need to do this a few times to become aware of how much firmer and stronger the legs are becoming. When you feel that the standing up of the long thighs gives the connection downwards of the feet into the earth, then walk with this awareness. It will need to be slow at first, but as you get into a rhythm you can speed up if you wish.

Can you feel the swing of your hips more now? We tend to walk from our knees, as our hips have become tight from sitting in chairs and car seats and holding ourselves 'together' at a feeling level. This puts strain on the knee joint and the thighs get very lazy, hence

the focus in this book on standing up through the thighbone. Can you feel the connection down of the feet towards the ground underneath you?

It would be good if you can sometimes walk on the earth barefoot, as this will help you feel the balance of the connection to the earth that gravity creates, and the lift off the earth, through the legs to the spine. We also have a tendency to push forward with the lumbar spine and the bottom of the breastbone, the sternum, especially if we are in a rush to get somewhere. The focus from the feet and legs lets the bottom of the sternum come back but lifts the top of the sternum towards the crown of the head. The spine is then aligned, as that will naturally bring the head up, and rest it back and down on the neck vertebrae. Doing this will have the effect of relaxing the shoulders out (2.4), rather than pulling them down, for then the upper back is hunched (2.5).

Shoulders respond to the movement of the hips. This is 'cross crawl'.

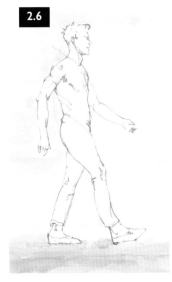

When the shoulders are relaxed, they naturally have a 'cross crawl' movement with the legs.

This does not come through trying to do it – the best action in which to feel it is crawling. It was in crawling as a child that you would have naturally first 'cross-crawled'. So come onto your hands and knees, and feel that as the left hand comes forward the right knee comes forward with it – or vice versa. Is it the knee or the hand that goes first? This is important as you will transfer this idea to walking when you come back onto your feet.

The next few paragraphs are from THE THINKING BODY, by Mabel Elsworth Todd.

'In the newborn infant, the spine is straight and very flexible, with all joints movable. The first muscles to attain power are those of the lumbar spine and pelvis, which the baby uses even before birth, squirming about, moving and straightening the lower back, drawing up the knees and throwing them out in the 'kick' familiar to all mothers....

'By much vigorous kicking and crying during the

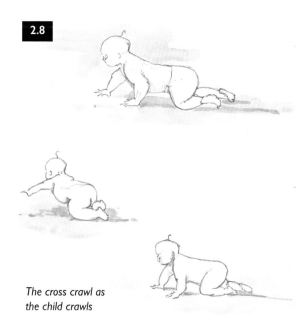

The cross crawl as the child crawls

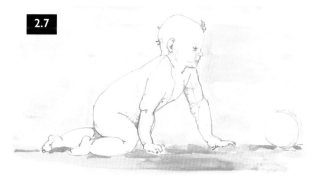

first months of its life, the baby develops those muscles which are needed to produce and stabilize the lumbar curve in its convex direction towards the front. Not until this curve has been established is the baby able to hold its head up, to sit or stand alone.

'The effect of the weight of the skull as the top-load is to produce another curve in the cervical region.

'Gradually the infant develops power in the minute muscles and ligaments about the vertebrae which control the secondary curves, by throwing his/her arms about, turning her/his head and lifting it while prone.

'Active movements and the resulting deeper breathing bring about the co-ordinated action of the entire spine. This process is greatly aided by spells of crying or screaming, since the diaphragm and the lower lumbar and pelvic muscles are so closely associated.

'In this way, by means of what may appear to be discomfort or distress, an axis of opposing curves is being established in the spinal column for the adequate support and movement of the body-weights. The head cannot be held up until this long axis is established. Power to sit, stand and walk comes only after this axis has been made secure by the strength of the deep spinal muscles and ligaments, whose intricate balancing action at the individual vertebrae has produced the opposing curves."

As the quotation makes clear, by the time we get

to crawling the spine is well prepared for the strong movement of the arms and legs, and then for the transition to standing with the so-beautiful upright spine that toddlers have and that we can regain.

When we crawled, we most likely did the movement of the hands and feet simultaneously. It is most helpful to look carefully at a crawling child or a four-legged animal – whenever you have one to hand! – so you can see the natural action that we hopefully once had (2.8). This is why it is most important not to try to ask a young baby to walk too soon; crawling is most important for the co-ordination of mind and body in later life.

Now you might find that you take the hands forward first; this is an indication of how much we move from the head and shoulders as we have become 'all up in

Crawling naturally leads to lifting up gradually through the legs and hips to standing (2.9 - 2.13)

2.9

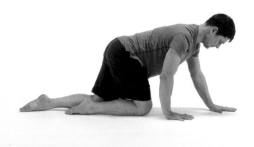

2.10

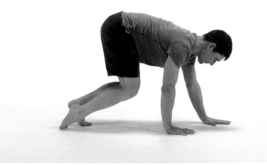

our heads' to the extent that we tend to drag the rest of the body around with our head! Can you consciously now move from the legs and let the hands and shoulders follow that movement?

If crawling is too much for you, then picture doing it in your imagination, or better still look at a baby crawling. What a wonderful movement! You will find that crawling babies often move very fast.

If we come back now to walking, can you feel how the movement of the lower body to the waist is counterbalanced by the upper body, so that there is a swing of the shoulders and arms as the legs swing through? Feel how this gives such a wonderful freedom of movement – it might make you want to dance!

Walking meditation

Walking (as we saw) has long been a way to process, understand and settle all that goes on in the mind. Consider how many times you have felt the need to go out for a walk when worldly cares seemed to press down on you. As we have seen, the rhythm of the movement when you stride out shifts and sorts the dilemmas the mind gets itself into.

To process them in walking, you do not need to think consciously about them all, indeed it is better not to. First of all, focus on the movement of your whole body, and feel your feet on the earth. It is much better to be directly on the earth – concrete has no give in

2.11

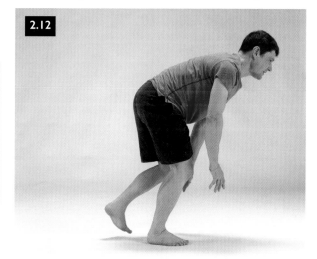

2.12

it, so that the feet, especially the arches, cannot work to support us, and then the spine and diaphragms are not as free to move. On concrete, we have to hold ourselves together more and then cannot breathe from the diaphragms.

Become aware of the movement of the spine in relation to the legs and feet, and feel all your toes aware of the earth underneath them. Feel the head sitting on top of the erect spine, looking out into the world around you. See and hear the world around you, aware of its wonders and seasons. Become aware of how you are breathing as you walk; you may be holding your breath to concentrate? Can you focus on your breath without interfering with it, as it will then gradually find its natural rhythm, which will go with the rhythm of your walk? You cannot make this happen, however your attention will bring you back to what is natural for your body.

The process of sitting goes from a focus within (in Sanskrit, *dharana*), usually on the breath or a mantra, to a 'being present' to the world around you, *dhyana*. There is this same process or movement in walking from the movement of your body to the awareness of, and our connection to, nature around you.

When you return, be aware how the mind has relaxed and eased. Sitting for a few minutes would be good now, to go with this shift of consciousness.

Now turn to running (chapter 3), if you wish, or to sitting (chapter 4).

2.13

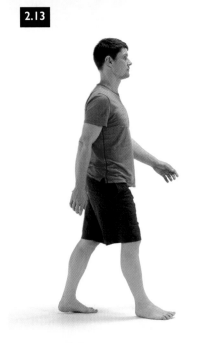

Chapter 3: Running

Patricia (Pachi) Lopez

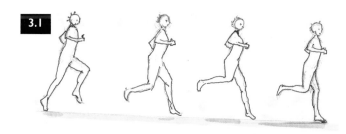

'The desire to run comes from deep within us – from the unconscious, the instinctive, the intuitive.' George Sheehan

Why running?

There are many reasons why we become runners. Some of the reasons people take up running are:

- To keep fit
- To lose weight
- To socialize
- For the enjoyment of being outside and in natural surroundings
- To get to know places
- To improve focus
- The challenge it offers
- To compete
- Low equipment cost compared with other sports
- Sense of achievement

Some run because it brings freedom and union between mind and body. For others, running can be an act of meditation.

Our ancestors developed the ability to run about four-and-a-half million years ago, probably in order to hunt animals. Today, even though we sustain this same ability, the use of running is totally different. Humans in the twenty-first century are mainly sedentary and not used to the strenuous movement of running. Outside of sport, we tend only to run when a part of our autonomic nervous system, the sympathetic nervous system (whose primary process is to stimulate the body's fight-or-flight response), is stimulated – for example, when we are in fear and need to run away from something or someone, or when we are afraid of missing a bus or train, and so on.

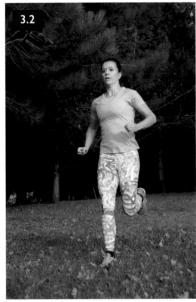

Choosing to Run

After we have mastered the art of walking, we can start integrating running into our practice if we so wish. Running doesn't differ much from walking, the only difference being the strength our body needs to speed up, lift more and overcome the increased external forces – for when we walk or run we have to overcome two elements of resistance: gravity and air. Gravity pulls us down and places a great force on our bones and joints. The greater our body mass, the greater the force coming down onto our bones and joints, too. In order to overcome gravity and the mass of air that we shift from in front of us as we run, the body needs to be stable and balanced. When running we also need to absorb shock during take-off and landing. Our ability to be aware becomes really important.

Running, just as does standing or walking, starts from the feet. The feet need to have free movement and be connected with the earth beneath. When we run we mistakenly tend to come down with the heel of the foot first, instead of the ball of the foot. The movement of bringing the foot forward should start

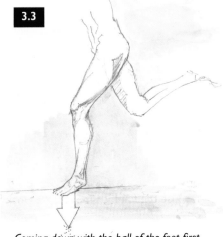

Coming down with the ball of the foot first

at the hip (3.2, 3.3), but this 'heel strike' comes from moving the knee and not engaging the hips. If we heel strike we are putting tension in our knees and our hips and we are stopping ourselves from going farther and quicker as we come down to the floor. We are not allowing ourselves to be helped by gravity, which works along with our upward movement from the earth to move us upwards and forwards.

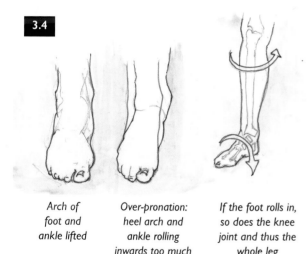

3.4

Arch of foot and ankle lifted

Over-pronation: heel arch and ankle rolling inwards too much

If the foot rolls in, so does the knee joint and thus the whole leg

Another important reason to land on the ball of the foot is to use the full foot movement when the foot lands on the floor.

Because we tend today to sit for very prolonged periods, the adductor muscles become lazy. This is one

of the reasons why the foot's inner heel drops (3.4, middle and right).

The action of the heel rolling inward or dropping as weight is transferred from it to the front foot is what we know as pronation. A certain amount of this is natural, but in many people the foot rolls in too much – that is, we overpronate.

In overpronating, the inward movement is exaggerated. With time this increases the stress on the muscles, tendons and ligaments of the foot and lower leg, including the shin and the knee, as the leg rotates in too far. Overpronation can cause injuries such as shin splints, plantar fasciitis (jogger's heel) and achilles tendonitis, as well as knee injuries. Connecting across the ball of the foot from the little toe joint to the big toe joint, as explained in the walking chapter, is a key to strong, stable and free movement of the feet.

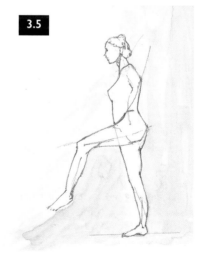

3.5

In the standing position (*tadasana*, see pp. 18-19 and 30-1), lengthen through your right foot and bring your left leg up, moving from your hip

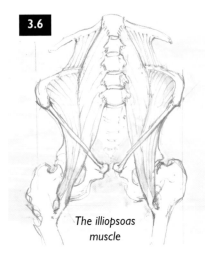

3.6

The illiopsoas muscle

(3.5). Feel how the action of moving from your hip, engaging the hip flexor muscles, will have an effect on your core. In this action the *illiopsoas* muscle (3.6), which we shall discuss in more detail on p. 50, is taking the leg up.

You should feel that both of your hips are level as you bring the leg up. The standing foot spreads on the floor beneath you, helping you to find balance. The thigh muscles should be relaxed and the foot should be in a neutral, dorsiflexed position as shown.

Now bring the left foot down in a controlled manner so that the hip flexors take the action. Feel how your foot will land on the ball rather than on the heel. Also feel how the foot lands right in line with the hip to allow the right foot to come up and follow the same process.

It is very important in running as it is a sagittal (one plane) movement (3.7) that comes from the mobility in the hips and pelvis, but we also need to stabilize these. From running being a repetitive movement, done in just one plane (thus sagittal), some of the stabilizer muscles of the hip and pelvis become weaker. That weakness of the hip stabilizers may be the cause of patelo-femoral pain and iliotibial band syndrome, both of which are common among runners.

Iliotibial Band Syndrome (ITBS) occurs when the iliotibial band, the ligament that runs down from the lateral part of the hip to the shin and stabilizes the outside of the knee as it flexes and extends (see Introduction, p. 12) is tight or inflamed. The pain is located on the outside of the knee and feels like a sharp pain that pulls the knee away.

The upper body and arms are key in the movement of running, but frequently they are neglected. The action of the arms will dictate how the legs move and not the other way around. Also holding a neutral spine where the sternum is lifted and the shoulders are relaxed helps you as a runner with your breathing.

Standing in *tadasana*, lift

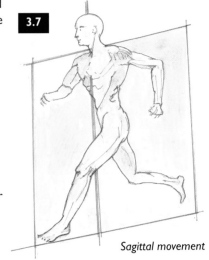

3.7

Sagittal movement

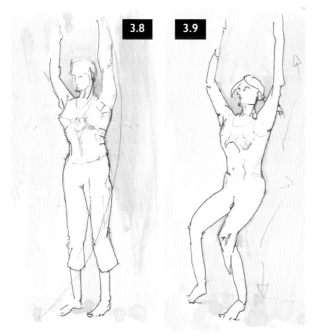

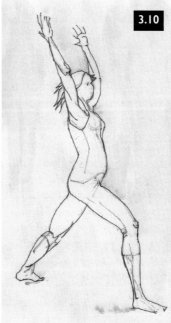

in the arm (3.8).

Repeat this movement so that you get familiar with the action of moving your arms from the *latissimus dorsi,* and the consequent retraction (a releasing movement down over the ribs) of the *scapulae* that this movement will bring, together with the sternum lifting. Now bend your knees, and feel that that takes you more into your legs (3.9). To lengthen your legs, come up through the

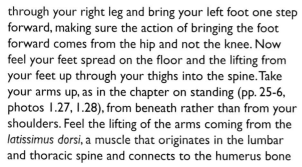

through your right leg and bring your left foot one step forward, making sure the action of bringing the foot forward comes from the hip and not the knee. Now feel your feet spread on the floor and the lifting from your feet up through your thighs into the spine. Take your arms up, as in the chapter on standing (pp. 25-6, photos 1.27, 1.28), from beneath rather than from your shoulders. Feel the lifting of the arms coming from the *latissimus dorsi,* a muscle that originates in the lumbar and thoracic spine and connects to the humerus bone

thighbone into the hip joint, connecting the feet down into the earth (3.8). This action should be taken into your running so that while you are running, your arm movement (from the muscles in your back) allows your shoulders to relax.

Now repeat the movement, and as your arms come up step your right foot forward, bending your right knee and keeping the lengthening of your left thighbone into the hip (3.10). The more you work on lengthening the right thighbone up into the hip joint, and coming forward and up through the left thighbone, the more you will feel the lifting of your sternum and a retraction down of your shoulderblades, allowing the heart and the diaphragm to open.

From *tadasana,* do the same with the other leg (3.10, 3.23-3.24).

It is important for the runner to work on the movement and lengthening of the spine, as the lumbar and cervical spine will stabilize the upper body and the thoracic spine will bring mobility, allowing the arms to move. Lack of self-awareness and the detachment of body from the mind are the reasons we tend to move by straining through the cervical spine rather than by opening the thoracic spine and so using the stronger, deeper back muscles below the neck, such as the *latissimus dorsi, multifidus* and *erector spinae,* which strengthen and lengthen the lumbar and thoracic spine. They in turn ease out the neck vertebrae – the cervical spine.

In the lumbar and cervical spine there are two natural curves in the structure (see pp. 25-6). These curves are like bridges, helping the whole structure of the body to be upright. The lumbar spine provides the connection of the lower body to the upper body, and through the lumbar spine we can feel the movement of the feet and legs. The support of the lumbar comes from the spread of the feet into the earth beneath us, which allows the bone structure of the legs to lift up into the hip bones supporting the pelvis, and which gives structure to the lumbar spine – enabling it to rest and lift at the same time as it stabilizes and supports the upper body. When there is a neutral (which is convex) curve in the lumbar spine and when the lumbar spine acts as a stabilizer of the body, the cervical spine can completely respond and come into its lesser neutral (convex) curve (1.18, 1.20)

The lumbar spine brings movement into the thoracic spine and helps the cervical spine to be the strong stabilizer for the head. The cervical spine is then capable of holding the head up and back into its atlas bone (1.19) again giving freedom to the thoracic spine, so that the shoulders can be relaxed and broad. When the body can perform in such a manner, when we find freedom in our posture and feel stable, then the body can run in the most natural way and for as long as it needs to.

Tree Pose

From standing position (*tadasana,* p. 31), lengthening through your right foot, bring the left knee up (3.11 left figure)

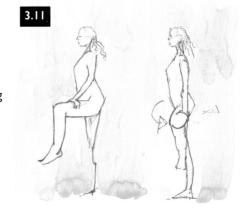

3.11

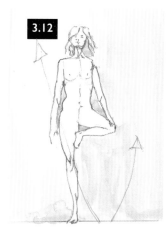

3.12

and hold it with your hand – making sure that the pelvis and hips are balanced. Now move the leg outwards and inwards and feel how the muscles around the pelvis and hips, *gluteus medius* and *minimus* engage on the movement and bring the foot down. Repeat on the other side.

Bring the left foot up again and take your to this pose. This is actually one of the regular yoga postures, tree pose (*vrksasana*, 3.16-21).

Practising tree pose you could feel how the spread of your standing foot puts you in contact with the floor beneath you as if your foot, especially your toes, are the roots of the tree spreading down into the earth giving the tree life and support. Standing in tree pose move your arms around before you bring them down and imagine what tree you could be in that moment (3.19, 3.20, 3.21).

For the body to be upright and for humans to be able to walk on two feet, we had to develop our core – this being the spine, the deep muscles of the abdomen (the *rectus abdominis* or ABS and the obliques), not

left heel and place it on your right inner thigh, keeping the lengthening through the right leg (3.12). Now feel how the stabilizer muscles of the hip and pelvis come into action – *illiopsoas, tensor fascia latae, rectis femoris* and *adductor longus* – allowing the pelvis and hip to be stable and balanced but bringing movement

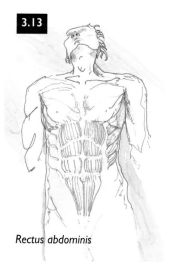

3.13

Rectus abdominis

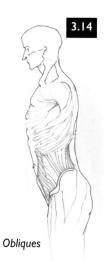

3.14

Obliques

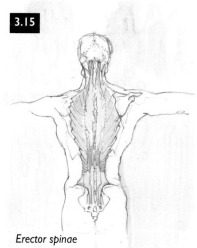

3.15

Erector spinae

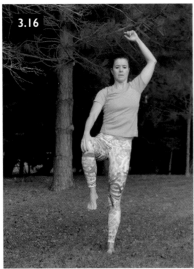
3.16

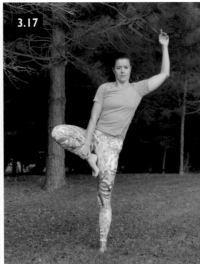
3.17

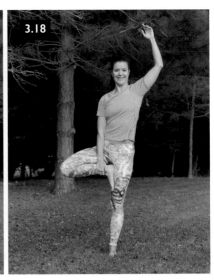
3.18

forgetting all the deep spinal muscles which maintain the whole structure.

A key muscle in the action of walking and running and the muscle that connects the lower with the upper body is the *illiopsoas*. You can see (3.6) that it connects from the inner leg to the iliac crest in the pelvis and also to the spine, as the *psoas* muscle.

The *illiopsoas* is considered a structural muscle but because of our lifestyle of sitting down most of the day on chairs and the lack of movement, this muscle has to function as a stabilizer in most people. This is all connected with the lack of strength in the stabilizer muscles such as the *multifidus* (see 1.20, 1.21), the

erector spinae (3.13, 3.15) in the back and the transversal abdominals and obliques (3.14) in the front of the body.

When these muscles are not engaged, the tendency of the upper body is to fall forward. We can see in a lot of runners that the shoulders are hunched forward, which will not only induce lower back pain but also limits the breathing, as the diaphragm movement is restricted. Standing again in *tadasana* (mountain pose, 1.11), your knees directly above your ankle joint (rather than braced back behind the ankle joint), your hips directly above the knees, then bend your knees forwards towards a squat, as though in a hinge movement.

Feel the spread of the feet on the floor beneath you,

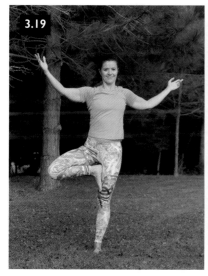
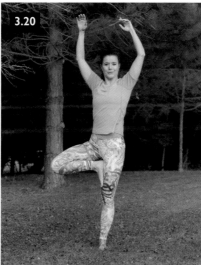
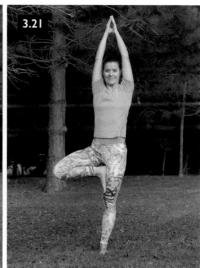

the connection of the big toe with your adductors and up to the groin and pelvis and the little toe connecting up the outer leg to the lateral edge of your hips. Come in and out of this posture by coming up through the thigh bone into the hip joint, opening the knee joint and bringing it back in line with the hips (see 3.8, 3.9). Now feel the *psoas* muscle from the top of your thigh up to your lumbar spine, the deep spine (*multifidus*) muscles bringing strength, and the strength continuing back up to the neck, forming the back of your core. Also feel the front muscles forming the core, and the *traversus abdomens* and obliques, which are engaged in this position.

Come back to *tadasana* (mountain) – only this time, when you bend your knees and hinge your hips, take your arms up, lifting them from beneath using your back muscles (*latissimus dorsi*) instead of your shoulders. Now feel how much this movement helps you in lifting from the lower back up to your neck and the thighs up to your sternum and how you then breathe from the thoracic diaphragm, opening the ribs.

Breathing

You may like to turn to the place in the chapter on standing where Jenny talks about breathing , pp. 29-31, and practise the 'tree of light' breath a few times, while also standing as she says. You would have read in that chapter that the way we can influence our breathing is by working on the body, but we cannot change the way we breathe just by practising breathing exercises.

The same is true when we run. Because we tend to run using our knees, our spine doesn't find the lengthening needing for it to lift up the sternum and the cervical spine and so stabilize the head.

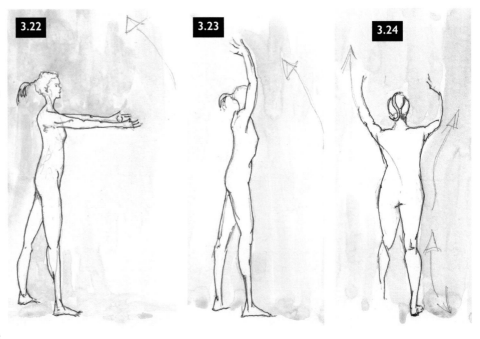

What happens when we don't lengthen through the spine is that we use the top of the lungs to breathe. Our diaphragm doesn't have the freedom to move and neither do we we take the breath from deep within us. Lifting up from *tadasana*, standing firm down through our feet, we can feel the breath coming from the pelvic diaphragm up to the thoracic diaphragm and finally come up to the throat diaphragm. This movement up from underneath the arms can make the arms want to come forward and up quite spontaneously, so that we then want to take a step forward (3.22, 3.23, 3.24).

When we breathe that way we can feel we are capable of taking more air in and out. We can also feel that our shoulders are able to relax and that the movement of the arms can really come from the feet rather than the shoulders – as we established before, when we spoke about the arms being lifted from beneath, using the *latissimus dorsi* muscles. Our body is sustaining us from the earth beneath us using our feet rather than allowing itself to be driven from our shoulders.

Another way we can practise the breath using the three diaphragms is with the help of mudras. Mudras (which, as we saw on pp. 10-11 are attitudes or gestures of consciousness) can be very helpful when running. In fact some elite runners use mudras as they run. For instance, a cue given to athletes when they run is to imagine they are holding a potato crisp between their fingers and they have to hold it carefully so it doesn't break. The symbol of holding the crisp is what we refer to in yoga as a mudra even though in the athletic world it is just a way to help you to relax your arms.

That opportunity is exactly what a mudra offers (3.25, 3.26). When you can practise the mudra while you are running, you can feel that your shoulders relax and your spine lengthens and that therefore your breathing is deeper too. Chapter 4 covers 'sitting', and you will find greater detail there, but you can get the feel of sitting right away to help you in running.

Find a way you can sit either on a chair or on the floor, somewhere you feel comfortable, but make

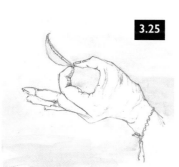

3.25

sure your spine is lengthened and that you feel the base spreading and the heart open. Now rest your arms on your thighs and bring the tip of the index finger to touch the tip of the thumb on each hand.

This is known as *gyana* mudra (3.25). Do you feel this gives the spread of the pelvic diaphragm as you inhale?

After a few breaths, take the index finger in to touch the first joint of the thumb (top picture 3.26).

Can you

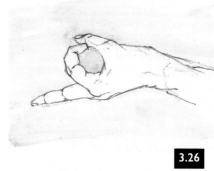

3.26

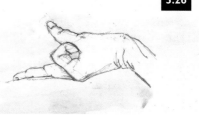

now feel this position of the fingers brings the opening of the thoracic diaphragm? After a few breaths, take the index finger in more to touch the root of the thumb (bottom picture 3.26).

Do you feel the movement of the throat diaphragm? The hand position with the index finger to the first and second joint is known as *chin* mudra. These mudras connect mind and body using the breath as a conscious connection.

You can also take the practice of *viloma* breathing (also known as the ladder breath, and given in Jenny Beeken's book, DON'T HOLD YOUR BREATH) into your running. Using this while you are running you can work on breathing in and out, as deep as you can go without forcing the breath.

For ladder breathing, pause as you inhale and then inhale again, so that the breath comes more deeply in, and then exhale. Do not hold the breath as you do this: it is a gentle, brief, pause only. Do that for two or three breaths. and then do the same on the exhalation. Exhale, pause – and at the end of the exhalation just let the breath come gently in. Again, do this two or three more times.

This *viloma* or ladder breathing can help you to find rhythm while you breathe. You may find that one pause on the inbreath and two pauses on the outbreath help you with your running. You may notice now that this ladder breath will help you breathe in and out more easily. The more you practise, the better you will get established and so feel more comfortable with your breath while running.

You need to know as well that the breath will change when your running speed changes, so you can adapt the breath to each situation.

Meditation

Meditation plays a big role in running. As we said before, some people run because in doing so they feel they can come within themselves; they feel they are in touch with what is happening inside their body and their mind. They are in total contact with both their body and their mind.

During running, we need to deal with a lot of mind chatter. One place where we are singularly inclined to this inner chatter is when running, and yet the more chatter in the mind the less you can focus on the run. This lack of focus is what makes a lot of people quit. Therefore if we practise the art of meditation and take it with us in our runs it will ease our way into the run and will allow us to stay with it for longer.

There are many ways of meditating and connecting to the part of us that is consciousness. We can focus our attention to our breath, use a mantra, or bring our awareness to the heart area of the body.

In the different stages of a run you may already find yourself doing any of these. You may be focusing on your breath, on telling yourself 'Yes, I can do this' (a mantra), or on pain in the physical body. However, when we do this we normally do it to fight the feeling that we are having in that given moment. We may be worried that our breath is too heavy and that we are not going to be able to carry on if we keep on breathing the same way. We may have a mind chatter telling us we cannot achieve the run, and silence it with a mantra telling ourselves 'we can do it'. Or we can just observe the pain in our physical body and analyze it.

When we come into meditation we look at the things that are going on in our body just as they are. We don't label anything, as we are only observers of what is happening within ourselves. When we are meditating and observing the breath, we only focus on the incoming air and outgoing air: we don't judge it as a breath, and therefore we are able to deepen into that breath and so ease the mind. It is the same with the chatter and the pain. If we don't judge it and don't label it we can feel and act beyond it.

One way of meditation which is very useful for runners is to sit still before you start and breathe into the different areas of your body, one after another. By doing this, when you are actually running you can take the consciousness with you and continue to meditate while you are running!

Sitting to Prepare for Running

Sit in a way that is comfortable to you, making sure that your spine is lengthening and that you are sitting on the base of the spine, lifting out from it to the crown during the whole meditation. Start by sitting for fifteen minutes and increase the time as you become more familiar with meditation, going up to as much as an hour.

Start with the thought of bringing your jaws away from each other so that your tongue can rest back and your cheeks can relax, and of bringing your eyes resting back from the eyelids so that they can roll back into their sockets and your brow can relax.

Now focus on your breath. Feel the air coming in and out of your nostrils. You can focus on the cool air touching your upper lip when the breath comes in and on the warm air when it comes out. After a couple of minutes you will already be feeling a sense of calm. Your mind may want to come into play and you may tend to engage with any thought that is coming to you. Rather

than staying with the thought or becoming irritated by it, take a deeper breath and observe it from a detached viewpoint and you will notice that the thought has dissipated. Another thought may then come into your mind, so you do the same process. While you are breathing more deeply observe that thought too, but try not to label it: again just observe it and observe that observing, and how the thought goes away when you focus back on your breath.

Now start bringing your breath towards your feet and your legs and breathe in and out of them. Observe all the sensation within the area, again trying not to label the feeling. Don't think, 'This is pain', 'This is pleasure': just observe it. When we label what we feel we are giving the instruction to the mind to feel good or bad about that feeling, but if we call all those feelings sensations we can treat them all the same way.

Keep on breathing in and out of your pelvis and sacrum, your back, your chest, your arms and hands.

While you breathe into each part of your body, explore the sensations around those areas. Observe how the sensations don't remain the same at any time. If you stop for a little bit longer to observe them, you can feel that the sensations are in constant change, that they don't remain the same – and by implication we can let them go and not cling onto them. There always comes a time where that sensation is going to pass away – and yes, another sensation is going to come in, but it is not the same one; it has already changed.

Now you are starting to wake up your consciousness and to be more aware of your true self.

The text that follows is based upon a talk given by Satya Narayan Goenka (Mr S. N. Goenka) in Berne, entitled THE ART OF LIVING: VIPASSANA MEDITATION.

'Breathing and sensations will help in two ways. First, they will be like private secretaries. As soon as a negativity arises in the mind, the breath will lose its normality; it will start shouting, "Look, something has gone wrong!" And we cannot scold the breath; we have to accept the warning. Similarly, the sensations will tell us that something has gone wrong. Then, having been warned, we can start observing the respiration, start observing the sensations, and very quickly we find that the negativity passes away.'

The more you practise this art of meditation when you are out running, and the more you become aware when your mind starts playing you up and you find all the chatter invading you, the better you are going to be able to find the balance you need in your body and mind. You will observe what is happening while you run, rather than just running. You should then be able to go on for longer and be in the moment throughout.

Chapter 4: Sitting

"I have seen in my wanderings great temples and shrines, but none are as blissful as my own body."
Mahasiddha Saraha, 8th century

SITTING, in the sense I mean it here, is a practice of being with ourselves as we are in the moment, in order to assess how we are, where we are and what is happening internally and/or externally, rather than sitting down to eat (although mindful eating is meditative), watch television, or be with friends. This practice of sitting (in the first sense) has long been a tradition in many societies, and we could call it 'meditation' even though our picture of meditation may be different. Wikipedia's definition of meditation is 'a practice in which an individual trains the mind or induces a mode of consciousness, either to realize some benefit or for the mind to simply acknowledge its content without becoming identified with that content or as an end in itself.'

Anybody who has sat with themselves even for one minute knows what an undertaking it is: just how identified with the mind's content we generally are. This passage from PERSON-CENTRED PSYCHOTHERAPIES by David Cain goes some way towards explaining this:

'Most of life is imaginary: human beings have a habit of compulsive thinking that is so pervasive that we lose sight of the fact that we are nearly always thinking. Most of what we interact with is not the world itself, but our beliefs about it, our expectations of it, and our personal interests in it. We have a very difficult time observing something without confusing it with the thoughts we have about it, and so the bulk of what we experience in life is imaginary things. As Mark Twain said: "I've been through some terrible things in my life, some of which actually happened".'

In India, it is traditional to sit at the feet of a person wiser than you, one known as a 'master', in order to listen to their wisdom. This is known in Sanskrit as *satsang*. Many thousands of people came to 'sit' and listen to the Buddha as well as many other yogis, and more recently to Ramana Maharshi and Krishnamurti. Many also came to hear such teachers as Pythagoras and Socrates in ancient Greece. We may also go to church to listen to a sermon, or to Buddha's monasteries to sit and listen to a *dhamma* talk. This is a particular type of sitting that focuses and trains the mind in listening, and it is an excellent step to meditation.

This chapter on sitting focuses the mind through the alignment of the body, and it could lead to meditation – but for the first several years it is helpful, I have found, to focus on alignment, posture, awareness and aliveness in the breath and body, and the present moment. For this reason I have called the chapter 'sitting', even though it addresses states of consciousness, as for many of us 'meditation' in all its many methods and ways of practice can feel too high and impossible an undertaking to a mind that as been over-stimulated in the intellect and so cut off from the intelligence and awareness of the body as well as the consciousness that is in the heart. It will also hopefully give a sense of the possibilities and introduce what is given in the ancient texts of such countries as India, China, Japan, Egypt, more particularly in the teaching of Buddha and Patanjali, as the text in this book relates more specifically to those teachings – to the extent that I believe I understand them.

Sitting in a Chair

When were chairs first introduced into western civilization? We see wonderfully upright statues of the Egyptian Pharaohs, whether by visiting somewhere such as the British Museum or going online (4.1). They sit so upright

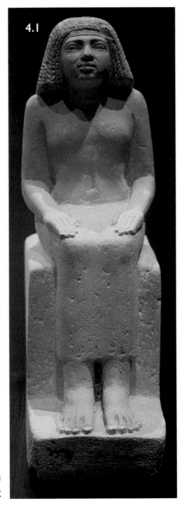

4.1

as they preside over their people.

Can we sit on a chair with this same upright spine, rather than slumped back and down in the chair as we so often see? Maybe yes, if the spine is now strong enough from our practice as we followed the standing, walking and maybe running chapters.

In many eastern countries people squat, rather than sit on a chair. This is wonderful for the arches of the feet, the hips and the spine: it keeps all of these alive and supple. One of my students told me that in Tokyo, at the train station, businessmen in their suits squat to read the newspaper as they wait for the train.

However, do not think of sitting in a chair as an easier option than sitting on the floor, as very important alignment of the legs and spine can be found with the chair. It is therefore good to practise this at some point even if you are used to sitting on the floor. Then you can also practise it when you have to sit on a chair in a waiting room, on a plane, on a bus or in a train. These situations are wonderful challenges, and doing this practice when you are obliged to wait can relieve feelings of impatience as well as keeping the body

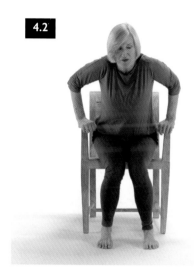

4.2

Getting up from a chair from the shoulders and arms creates strain in the neck, shoulders and upper back

and mind alive and connected. First of all notice how we tend to sit down in a chair and how we get up from our chair. Often we collapse heavily down and then push on the chair from the shoulders and arms to heave ourselves up again (4.2).

How can we stay with the awareness of our posture in standing and walking when we come to sit in a chair? Can we use the same principles of moving from the feet and legs to sit down and get up? This will take strain off the shoulders and arms. The chair needs to be upright and comfortable with the right support in the back if that is needed – although hopefully, after a while spent working on this, the support will not be needed. Do have a cushion or block, though, to support your back

to make it comfortable if you have any strain or pain.

Make sure the chair is not going to slip on a polished floor: it can be back against a wall if necessary. If you have strain in the shoulders your chair may need arms but see if you can stand up and sit down without using them, so that you do not put weight and strain into the shoulders but use the feet and legs as nature intended.

Sitting Down

With feet near the chair, take your arms forward to balance your weight, and stand evenly down. Spread down through your feet, but up and back through your thighbone and forward and up through your spine, so that you sit lightly down through the base of the spine.

Feel how your feet had to go firmly down into the earth to enable you to sit lightly down on the chair. And if you are aware of the base of the spine as it goes down, then the lumbar part of it lengthens up off the sacrum as in standing (chapter 1). The shoulders can then release and relax out to the side, in turn relaxing your hands by spreading them on your thighs. Make sure your ankle bone is directly below the knee joint and the knee joint is in line with your hips: you may need a block or book or two under your feet to do this if the chair is too high for you.

Now hold one wrist and take your arms forward to the level of your shoulders. Keeping your shoulders relaxed, go down through your feet as though you wanted to stand up. Feel the 'forward and up' length that that gives to the spine. Keep that length and let your arms relax back down, resting the spine back in one piece – this means moving the spine as one, rather than moving from the head and shoulders and taking the body with it, which is what we have tended to do, as we have become so head-orientated. Repeat, holding the other wrist (shown in 4.3 and 4.4).

Now bring your fingers around your kneecaps (4.5; if this pulls on your shoulder joint take your fingers higher up on your thighs) and lift one heel slightly off the ground. Feel the lift of your kneecap and shinbone into your hand, then keep that lift as you take the heel forward and down.

See if you can come down through the front of the heel before the back of the heel goes down, as this will engage the arch of the foot and the anklebone more. Feel how hard the lower leg and foot need to work to keep the lift. They need to be working like this all the time to support your whole body. But once you have engaged these deep postural muscles then it will gradually feel more natural (see the labelled drawing of the *tibialis posterior* in the standing section: 1.7).

If the shinbone is braced back then this vital postural muscle has become bowed back behind the ankle joint and therefore unable to do its job of standing straight up into the knee joint.

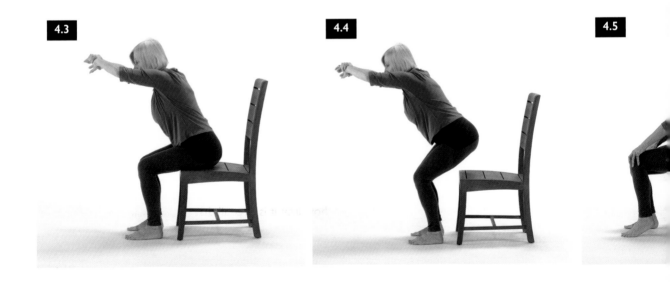

4.3 **4.4** **4.5**

Repeat on the other side.

Then put the left hand around the right kneecap and the right hand flat on the right side of the sacrum, with the fingers pointing down so that the spine is gently twisted on its axis to the right..

Repeating the lift of the heel, ease the hand around the kneecap, back towards hand on the sacrum, as though you want to fit the head of the femur deeper into the hip socket. Keep the right hand firm into the sacrum to help that movement – rather like easing the foot into a snugly-fitting shoe. Keep that movement on the thigh and shinbone as you take the heel back down. Can you feel how this lifts the spine, makes it more

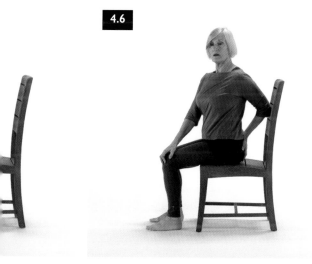

4.6

upright, and see how much the spine moves from the life in the legs and feet (4.6)? Repeat on the other side.

Standing Up

Feeling that standing up of the thighbone into the hip socket, take one wrist, again bringing the arms forward and up and the feet firmly down, to stand straight up off the chair (the pictures for sitting down, 4.3 and 4.4, equally apply to standing up). Do not brace the knees back, as Michael is doing with his left knee in 4.7, above, but rather lift the thigh off the knee joint as I am doing in 4.8. Change the hold of the wrist and sit lightly back down. Feel how light it is after all that waking up of your legs and feet! You can repeat this several times, sitting down

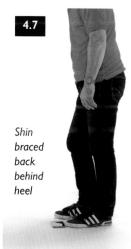

4.7

Shin braced back behind heel

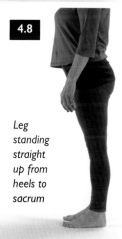

4.8

Leg standing straight up from heels to sacrum

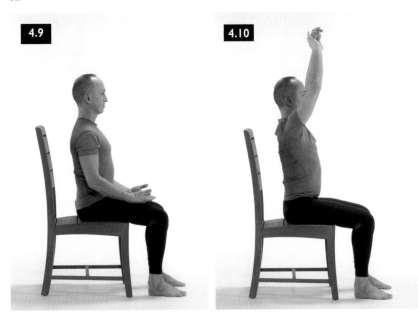

If you feel the spine collapses back at any point, bring the arms forward and up (4.10) so the spine returns to its alignment of the base and the crown. You can now either go on into meditation (see the section beginning p. 65), or to sitting on the floor.

Sitting on the Floor

There are many different postures for sitting on the floor and you can move around from one to the other to see which one works for you in the particular moment. This may change over time. It is most important to have the spine aligned, the crown above the base.

more lightly and easily each time. Feel now as you sit that your feet can really spread down and engage with the ground underneath them, which has the effect of engaging the whole length of your legs up and back into their hip sockets.

The spine then responds to this engagement of the legs and feet by lengthening forward and up.

Feel how you now sit straight up through the length of the spine to the crown of the head, as Thierry is doing in photo 4.9). Stay sitting like this, aware of your spine and aware of your breath.

I find it useful to free up my hips with yoga postures, but first by sitting for a moment on my knees, with the heels very active, lifting in and up (4.11).

This has the effect of elongating the spine up off the pelvis so that it is not heavily down on the feet. This is called *vajrasana* in Sanskrit, which means either 'thunderbolt pose' as if the feet are very active (and then the spine moves strongly forward and up) or 'diamond' pose, as there is a deep pointed connection in the base, then a broadening out across the thoracic diaphragm, and

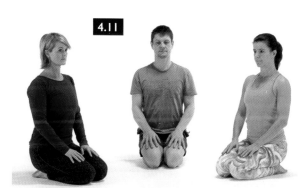

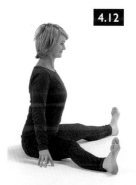

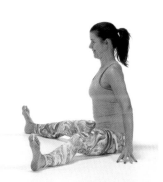

Vajrasana (thunderbolt or diamond pose)

Upavistha konasana

so a coming to a point at the crown of the head.

This feeling may not last long, so then move to the wide angle pose (*upavistha konasana*) then cobbler (*baddha konasana*). These two poses will enable you to sit with freer hips and a more upright spine now in a cross-legged pose – *parvatasana* – literally mountain pose.

Upavistha konasana *(wide angle pose)*

Sit on the base of your spine with the legs out, comfortably wide, but not too wide, as the inner and outer legs need to be aligned with one another, so that the kneecaps are facing upwards towards the ceiling. If your knees or hips are under any strain, then let the knees bend up and even take the feet on the floor as this will bring more life to the feet (the hips and knees are

usually under strain because the feet are not working to support us).

Take your fingertips onto the floor as in 4.12, Anchor down into your heels so the legs connect back into the the hip joint, and then gather back from the toetips and fingertips, through all the joints, to the spine, so that you feel the spine comes forward and up in alignment.

When you have felt that, bring your feet together into *baddha konasana*.

Baddha konasana *(cobbler pose)*

Rest out through your legs, and then spread the heels and balls of the feet into one another to gather back through the knees, hands around the knees as shown (4.13, overleaf), so that the knees come slightly towards

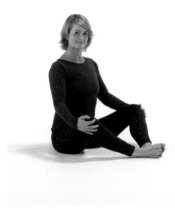

4.13

Baddha konasana, caught angle pose (cobbler pose)

one another and back to the thighs. Feel what happens to the spine when you do that. Does it align forward and up from the base of the spine?

This can be a comfortable pose in which to sit against the wall with a cushion or block at the level of the sacrum and the hands resting on the knees. Or go on to *parvatasana*.

Parvatasana (mountain pose)

In *parvatasana*, the mountain, you are aligned like a mountain with your peak towards the heavens. Take one foot under the opposite knee so that it comes into line with the opposite hip and the other foot is in line with the opposite knee, making a square shape (4.14).

This will bring the spine into alignment but is demanding on the hips, so you may not be able to stay long at first. That is fine, because in a second or two of

total focus you can feel more connected to the divine in you than after hours of struggle.

Anchor down into the little toe, rest out through the knees, and then gather back from the soles of the feet to the spine. Feel how the hips open and free up as the spine comes forward and up, so that the head then sits up and back on top of the neck vertebrae, so that the crown is in line with the base.

This alignment relaxes the mind down naturally so there is a connection between the mind and body. The jaw, eyes and brain all then relax back and down physically. This is then a body-centred sitting already, and the best place to begin 'sitting' in the deeper sense. You can spend some time with this awareness of the connection and oneness of the body and mind first, however.

The *hasta* mudras can also help relaxation and focus

4.14

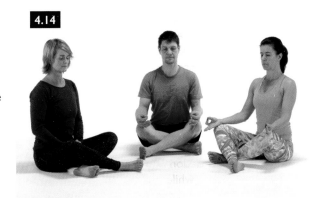

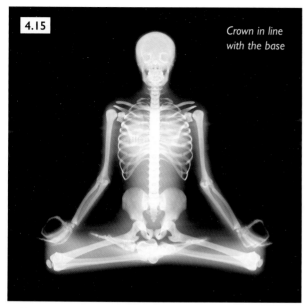

4.15

Crown in line with the base

as long as the hands are relaxed.

If the hands are on the knees with the palms turned upwards the fingers spread out and form a gentle upturned dome back into the palm. The *palma fascia* is a strong tendinous muscle, which is the hand's counterpart to the *plantar fascia* in the foot, the muscle that helps create the arch. At a subtle body level these are both chakras (energy centres). Also, the awareness tends to be going outwards and bringing a natural easy deepening of the inhalation and the exhalation.

If the palms, after a while of sitting, are then brought into the lap **with the left** hand in right for a man and the right hand in the left for a woman, this then brings the focus more into the centre of your being and the breath settles to its normal rate but keeps the natural rhythm that the deepening of your breathing gave.

Meditation

After developing our awareness in standing, walking and running, and in the body instructions for sitting, we might then feel ready to address what happens to the mind when we 'sit' with all of this awareness. (Equally we might not, and that is fine: standing and walking and running, practised in this mindful way, also have a profound effect on the mind, bringing clarity and calm.)

As soon as we relax into our awareness of mind, we tend to become aware that the mind is constantly chattering, just as Patricia has extensively described happening in running. If we can be aware of that, and observe it, then we realize that the mind is not the sum total of who we are, because we can be aware of what it is doing. What then is this awareness and where is it?

Are we consciousness, defined as 'the quality or state of awareness, or of being aware of an external object or something within oneself'? This is a rather mundane description, but the mind also has the ability to expand beyond the limitations of the physical body. It can travel out to feel the stars, the birds, the universe, and connect across the oceans to loved ones, if we will but let it and trust this ability within us.

Meditation consists of connecting to ourselves that

part of us that is consciousness, wholeness, oneness. It also means realizing that the mind is not essentially the sum total of who we are. As in the words from THE YOGA SUTRAS OF PATANJALI at the end of the introduction, what we are is pure unbounded consciousness.

The initial way to feel this consciousness is to be aware that we can witness what the mind is doing with its busy chatter, so if we can witness it, then it is not us – for who is witnessing it? This is called witness consciousness. The Buddha called it *vipassana,* which means 'seeing things as they really are'.

The quantum physicist Dr John Hagelin, in a YouTube interview with Russell Brand, describes modern science in a particular way. He explains how, since Albert Einstein, physicists have been looking for a unified field of consciousness, and that this is what the super string theory offers. Once found, it would state that all of life is consciousness and all the things that exist are ripples on the consciousness. This, he reminds us, is what we touch when we meditate.

Ken Wilber, in one of his deep and delving books, called THE SPECTRUM OF CONSCIOUSNESS, considers that what we call consciousness is actually a spectrum, with ordinary awareness at one end and a more profound type of awareness towards the other. He likens this to the electromagnetic spectrum:

'Our environment is saturated with numerous kinds of radiation – besides the common visible light of various colours, there exist x-rays, gamma rays, infrared heat, ultraviolet light, radio waves, and cosmic rays.

'All of these radiations are superficially quite different from one another. x-rays and gamma rays, for instance, have very short wavelengths and consequently are very powerful, capable of lethally damaging biological tissues; visible light, on the other hand, has a much longer wavelength, is less powerful and thus rarely harms living tissue. From this point of view they are indeed dissimilar. As another example, cosmic rays have a wavelength less than a millionth of a millionth of an inch, while some radio waves have a wavelength of over a mile. At first glance these phenomena all seem to be radically different.

'However, all of these radiations are now viewed as different forms of an essentially characteristic electromagnetic wave, and are simply described as being different bands of one spectrum.'

Wilber goes on to compare this with Lama Govinda's description of consciousness being composed of several shades, bands or levels.

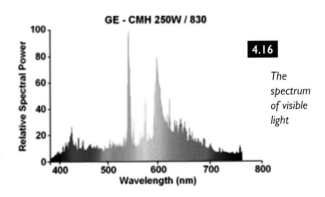

4.16

The spectrum of visible light

'Govinda states that these levels "are not separate layers … but rather in the nature of mutually penetrating forms of energy, from the finest all-radiating, all penetrating, luminous consciousness down to the densest form of 'materialized consciousness', which appears before us as our visible, physical body"'.

So consciousness, like electromagnetic radiation, is there within us all and around us, all of the time. We can 'touch in' to consciousness or awareness at any moment; we do not need to spend our life sitting and trying to feel it. The most spiritual life is an ordinary one lived in the world as it is, but touching into this spectrum of consciousness at any time. To do so makes an enormous difference as to how we then live our life.

At this present time 'mindfulness' is a buzz word and the practice of mindfulness is taught in many ordinary places such as hospitals, workplaces, businesses. This is a wonderful development, yet I have heard the Abbot, Ajahn Sucitto, at the Cittaviveka Theravada Buddhist Monastery, in Chithurst, West Sussex, in a Dhamma talk, ask: 'Why has only mindfulness been taken, somewhat out of context, from the Buddha's vast teaching; why not compassion, virtue, loving kindness, equanimity and the rest?'

The more we touch into what the Abbot terms 'heart consciousness', the more we will live our life mindful of these broader principles and be able to put them into practice in our daily life. So although we might practice 'mindfulness' in our daily lives or as a meditation practice, we can be aware of the vastness of the very ancient teaching that it encompasses so

encouraging that awareness of the qualities that are within us all that can come out of the practice of mindfulness.

So what is heart consciousness? Jesus Christ says, 'Love one another; as I have loved you' (John 13:34). Isn't this heart consciousness? He also said, 'I and my Father are one' (John 10:30) and 'That they all may be one; as thou, Father, art in me, and I in thee, that they also maybe one in us.... I in them, and thou in me, that they may be made perfect in one....' (John 17:21-23)

Isn't this Christ consciousness, too, if Christ consciousness is defined – as it is by the Florida-based Center for Christ Consciousness – as 'the growing human recognition and blending of the human evolutionary (or ego) mind with the Divine Mind'?

The teacher White Eagle says,

'Life is consciousness; as a being grows and evolves he or she is expanding individual consciousness. The extent of a human being's spiritual power is the extent of his or her consciousness of higher realms of life, the conscious acceptance of new heights and depths and breadths of a fuller, richer and more abundant life.

'So, in the degree that you become more conscious of the smallest details both in human life and in the world of nature, so you will begin to expand, grow and evolve in consciousness.

'This expansion depends however entirely upon your individual reactions to life.

'For every experience small or great, sweet or bitter, is intended to give you a further opportunity to expand your consciousness.'

White Eagle is also here putting the emphasis on respect for life in all its aspects and how we live our lives in the world. In this way we retain the wonder of life in all its many forms.

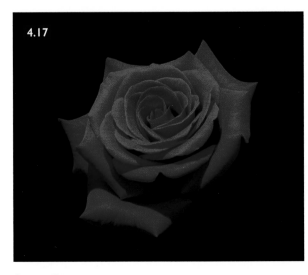

4.17

Samadhi

Let us return to the concept of 'witness consciousness', which means standing a little outside of ourselves to get some awareness of what might be going on: not to analyze or even understand on an intellectual level but just to witness. Once we have witnessed our thoughts, then we can go beyond them to the unified field of consciousness or heart consciousness, or to the absolute, the unmanifest – which is termed *Brahman* in the ancient Vedic tradition that underlies Hinduism and yoga. In one form or another, this concept is there in all the mystical traditions of all the world's religions. Cosmic consciousness is found when we have touched into the oneness of all beings, the oneness of the whole universe, and beyond this universe into the Cosmos. This is a stage of meditation in both yoga teaching and the Buddha's teaching, in both called *samadhi*, which can be translated as oneness with all life, total absorption, or one-pointed concentration.

This awareness of oneness may exist only for an instant, but once we have touched this field nothing will ever be the same again to us. For we become aware that we are not a collection of our thoughts and feelings: rather, we know that there is an awareness beyond this self – a self that has to function in the day-to-day world – and yet the day-to-day world is still the place wherein we can be aware of that awareness!

Notice how we feel when we see a beautiful sunset, a tree coming into leaf, a new born baby, or when we witness someone close to us die. We often easily and naturally make a contact with this unified field of consciousness then, but it is there all the time for us in any instant, not just in moments of crisis. When we make a conscious decision to sit with ourselves as we are, we are in touch with that unbounded field of consciousness. We might not feel this for the whole time, as the thoughts overshadow that field, but it is there.

This is why meditation is so energizing and uplifting, even when thoughts come in a lot, because we have seen them for what they are: not the essence of ourselves but a ripple on the surface of our consciousness.

There are different ways to touch this consciousness. The first stage of meditation, *dharana,* mentioned in chapter 2 – the chapter on walking, where we discussed how we can focus on the movement of the body, from our feet and legs, and how their movement connects us to the spine, and regard this as *dharana.* The most literal translation of *dharana* is 'bringing the mind to bear on…'. In sitting *dharana* is to focus the mind on an object such as our breathing, a mantra, or the heart and breath area of the body.

In standing and walking and in our sitting posture we have focused on the alignment of the base of the spine area and the crown area; then when we sit in meditation we can come to the centre of this axis, which is the heart area – heart consciousness is literally focusing our gaze and so our mind down to the heart centre in the centre of the chest, as the breath comes and goes.

The physical heart, which is felt slightly to the left of centre of the chest area, has long been a source of interest and fascination as it is responsible for pumping the blood around the body. It is directly connected to the lungs, and full movement of the lungs from the diaphragms of the body massages the heart and so keeps it healthy. There is also an energy centre at the level of the physical heart on the axis of the spine which is called the heart centre. In Sanskrit this is the *anahata*

chakra – where *anahata* means 'unstruck sound' and *chakra* means wheel or vortex of energy.

There are direct connections from the heart to the brain, and it has long been thought that the brain controls the heart. Recent discoveries, however, show that there are far more neural pathways from the heart to the brain than the other way around. What is the implication of this?

On the level of conscious practice there is the seeking of heart consciousness. This is taking our focus away from the head, brain and mind area and bringing it down to the heart area. This settles the mind, gives us a much more expanded awareness of ourselves, others and the world around us, and also brings an awareness of the rhythm of the breath moving through our body. It is a practice of giving the 'heart mind' precedence over the mind in the head and is a very essential focus for meditation.

Some recent research on the heart is discussed in the book THE EMOTION CODE by Dr Bradley Nelson (the emphasis is Dr Nelson's own):

'Your heart generates 60 to 1000 times more power and electromagnetic energy than your brain, easily making it the most powerful organ in your body. When you were in the womb, your heart was formed first, before your brain. Your heart beats about 100,000 times a day, 40 million times a year, and if its connection to your brain was severed, it would keep right on beating.

'Your heart is the core of your being, the core of who you really are.

'New research shows that your heart is much more

than a mere pump. In the 1970s scientists learnt that
the heart has an elaborate nervous system, a discovery
that has led to the creation of a new branch of
medicine known as neurocardiology. The fact is, we all
have two brains.

'Much to these scientists' surprise, they discovered
that the brains in our head are *obeying* messages sent by
the "brains in our hearts".

'Your heart is constantly sending out information
to your body. Every beat carries critical messages that
affect your emotional and physical health.

'**The heart has its own unique intelligence. It can
think, feel and remember.**

'**When you feel love toward someone, you are
actually sending out a powerful electromagnetic
signal to them, using the heart brain.**'

So in meditation, when we relax our awareness
physically and mentally down to the heart and breath
area, the mind in the head begins to settle into
the oneness of being. This is *samadhi*. To relax our
awareness in this way we must keep the alignment of
the crown of the head above the base of the spine, as
then there is a physical connection through the nervous
system of the body. If this is not physically possible from
some disability in the body it can still be energetically
possible by focusing the mind down to the heart and
visualizing that alignment.

The brain sits at the top of the spinal column and
connects the heart and the rest of the body via the
spinal cord (4.18). If there is some restriction caused
by the head being too far forward, then the settling of

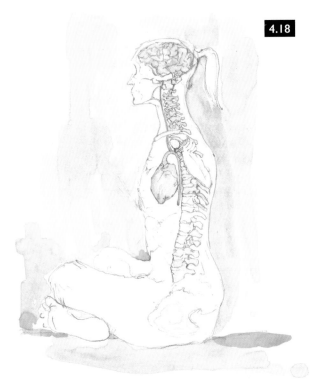

4.18

mind has no chance of being maintained – so when you
are aware that the mind has gone off on a topic (which
it will constantly do, that is its nature: we are not trying
to stop it, which is impossible, but we can become
aware that the wandering is not the sum total of our
being), just come back to the alignment of the spine, the
connection all the way up from the feet to the crown of

the head, and then feel what happens to the busy-ness of the so-called monkey mind.

This is the struggle for the psyche. It is defined, from the psychological point of view, as 'the totality of the human mind, conscious and unconscious'. However, when we look at the etymology, we find that the basic meaning of the Greek word *psyche* was 'life' in the sense of 'breath', to be summed up as 'self in the sense of the conscious personality' (both these definitions are from Wikipedia). This makes it clear to me somehow that the psyche is of this life, of the breath that we breathe in this body, whereas the consciousness that we can touch, become aware of, in our practice (defining practice as any action that lets us become aware of consciousness) is beyond the personality, beyond an individual life, beyond time and place. It exists everywhere, forever, outside of time and space.

Dharana and Dhyana

However there are many times when we feel lost and caught up in worldly worries and cannot feel that we are contacting anything so profound. It is essential, for instance, never to be attached to 'having a good experience' when sitting. Some meditations have even been described as 'shopping list' experiences. This wide range of awareness is a recognized stage of meditation and is accounted for in the stage of meditation that follows *dharana*. This second stage is *dhyana*, sometimes translated both as contemplation and meditation in itself.

To me *dhyana* encompasses all that happens when we engage in this enormous undertaking to sit and be with ourselves. *Dharana* is the intention and the act of sitting, focussing, lighting a candle, repetition of a mantra, and *dhyana* is what comes out of that intention: the awareness that it gives of the whole of our self and the world around us. This is enormous and can be overwhelming in its entirety. Can we stay with that entirety without getting absorbed into any one part of it? This is the vastness of being human that *dhyana* – awareness, contemplation – puts us in touch with.

When we become aware we have gone on to our shopping list (and it is often worries, fears about the future or regrets and resentments about the past) then we have a choice.

We can either come back to *dharana*, focusing the mind on the breath, the mantra, the present moment: the sound of birds, the earth underneath us, a candle, a beautiful view; or we can stay with *dhyana* to reflect or contemplate what comes up in the mind so that the mind chatter is then transformed into a profound reflection of our life, our thoughts, our whole process of being.

We may see a pattern, a tendency, a moving through, even – so this is a cycle. It is awareness of this cycle without getting caught up in it, being able to let it be, almost a feeling of literally going beneath it to the level of the heart centre: that is my understanding of *dhyana*. It can take us to faith in ourselves that we are in some way being guided, taken care of, by some inner awareness or being; we only need listen to this inner awareness and have the courage to act on it in our lives. So we move in our minds between the focus of *dharana* and the reflection of *dhyana* – and maybe within that process touch for an instant an opening, a clarity, an understanding of the wholeness of our being: an at-one-ment with the world around us. This is the way to *samadhi* – it is a glimpse of enlightenment of a true reality of our being.

Be aware that the our image of our self, our ego sense, known as *ahamkara* in Sanskrit, will resist this practice. This experience of sitting, and what surfaces in that endeavour, can be very overwhelming and we do try to resist it. Regular meditation is really going to change our perspective of who we are and will bring many inner changes. The psyche will resist these changes. The Buddha called this 'clinging', and stated that it is the cause of our suffering.

Michael A. Singer, in his book, THE UNTETHERED SOUL, which I highly recommend for all those struggling in meditation (which we all of us are, one way or another!) says

'When you are lost and struggling with all these psychological changes, you are suffering. In truth the very responsibility of having to hold it all together is a form of suffering.

'In order to understand clinging, we must first understand who clings. As you go deeper into yourself, you will naturally come to realize that there is an aspect of yourself that is always there and never changes. This is your sense of awareness, your consciousness. It is this

awareness that is aware of your thoughts, experiences the ebb and flow of your emotions and receives your physical senses. This is the root of Self. You are not your thoughts; you are aware of your thoughts. You are not your emotions; you feel your emotions. You are not your body; you look at it in the mirror and experience this world through eyes and ears.'

This reminds me of the principle of the three gunas from the *Bhagavad Gita* – here from the translation by Swami Prabhavanda and Christopher Isherwood:

'The Gunas are that in us which compels us to act:

Rajas – that which compels us to do, to achieve, to make happen. Tamas – that which binds us, preventing action creating dullness. Sattwa – that which uplifts to joy, lightness, happiness.'

'Rajas the passionate will make you thirsty for pleasure and possession:

'Rajas will bind you to hunger for action.

'Tamas the ignorant bewilders all men.

'Tamas will bind you with bonds of delusion.

'Sattwa can show you the Atman by its pure light: yet sattwa will bind you to search for happiness.

'When sattwa prevails over rajas, tamas

'Man feels that sattwa:

'When rajas prevails over sattwa, tamas,

'Man is seized by that rajas:

'When tamas prevails

'Over rajas, sattwa,

'Man yields to that tamas.

'A man is said to have transcended the Gunas when he does not hate the light of sattwa, or the activity of rajas, or even the delusion of tamas while these prevail; and yet does not long for them after they have ceased.'

We might feel that we have very little control over our actions and our lives, so that the principle of these gunas can seem to give us license to be ruled by the compulsion in us to act or not. But again what is needed is awareness of these energies within us that can be so compelling.

Dhyana can be reflection on actions that are in our past or those that we contemplate in the future; this will enable us not to be so pulled in these different directions the gunas can appear to impose on us.

We can recognize here the ups and downs, the different phases we have in our lives and in our minds. Meditation is allowing those phases to be as they are: a necessary part of our understanding of our psyche that allows to go beyond it to our true eternal Self, known as the *Atman* in yoga. The *Atman* is one with and part of *Brahman*; *Brahman* is pure unbounded consciousness or cosmic consciousness.

This is what we are grappling with in meditation: seeing the conscious personality for the changeable, susceptible, limited part of us and touching the beyond, the Spirit, unbounded consciousness. Constantly in our endeavours to sit with all of this we go between the two. This is allowed for in *dhyana*, the second stage of meditation.

We might sit for twenty minutes (a good time length of time to begin with) and touch such consciousness for an instant, and some days apparently not at all.

No matter: it is our intention to sit and be with ourself that is important, not what we judge to be the result, or what happens in that time. This is an enormous undertaking for minds that have been trained to be so active and busy, so we need to 'just do it' and not judge ourselves in it.

You will gradually feel what an enormous difference this makes to you in daily life, and in your interactions with the world, nature, and those you come into contact with including the plant and animal world – and of course those who are dear to you.

The next quotation is intended to give you some idea of the enormousness that contemplation can put you in touch with. It is again from the Yoga Sutras of Patanjali. Not much is known about Patanjali – we do not even know if he was one person or several – but he is known as the 'father of yoga' and is said to have lived at the time of the Buddha. He would have most likely gone to hear the Buddha teaching and maybe was one of those renowned yogis who debated with the Buddha.

In the system of yoga associated with Patanjali there are what are known as 'limbs', eight of them in all. The first two of the eight limbs of yoga are the groundwork of our living, while our practice of the second six enables us to put these very challenging principles into practice. The quotation overleaf is from THE YOGA SUTRAS OF PATANJALI, in the translation by Alistair Shearer:

'2.29 There are eight limbs of yoga:
Yama – the laws of life
Niyama – the rules for living
Asana – the physical postures
Pranayama – awareness of breath
Pratyahara – the retirement of the senses
Dharana – the steadiness of mind
Dhyana – meditation
Samadhi – the settled mind.
'2.30—The laws of life are five:
Non-violence
Truthfulness
Integrity
Chastity or continence
Non-attachment.
2.31—these laws are universal. Unaffected by time, place, birth, or circumstance, together they constitute the "Great Law of Life".
2.32—The rules for living are five:
Simplicity
Contentment
Purification
Refinement
Surrender to the Lord.
2.35—When we are firmly established in nonviolence, all beings around us cease to feel hostility.
2.36—When we are firmly established in truthfulness, action accomplishes its desired end.
2.37—When we are firmly established in integrity, all riches present themselves freely.
2.38—When we are firmly established in chastity, subtle potency is generated.
2.39—When we are firmly established in non-attachment, the nature and purpose of existence is understood.'

In these sutras, nos. 2.29–2.32 give guidelines for living earthly life, while sutras 2.35–2.39 give the wonderful and amazing effects of living by these guidelines. These effects need much contemplation – *dhyana* – to grasp what they encompass and where we can be in our whole consciousness. They correspond in some way to all the religions of the world: to the Ten Commandments of the Bible, which are encompassed by Judaism , Islam and Christianity; to Jesus Christ's teaching; and the Buddha's eightfold path and five precepts.

As we deepen a regular practice of anything from a minute's contemplation of the world around us to hours of meditation, yoga or practice in whatever path we are drawn to, and retain a continuing awareness or mindfulness of how we live our lives – including how we walk, stand and sit, run, or whatever way we choose to move our body – we can see that we are travelling towards these principles. Maybe it seems we move slowly, with some apparent backward steps, but in terms of the cosmos of many millions of years our lifespan on earth is infinitesimally short. So we need tremendous patience with ourselves and all others that we interact with to come to a magnanimous place of being in this world as it is right now.

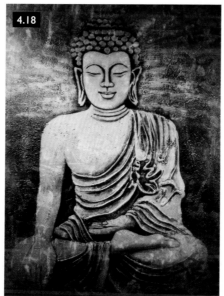

4.18

This way of being can be criticized for being too passive when there are so many problems and so many people living in dire poverty, displaced from their homes, and so much cruelty and fighting. However it has been shown, as in Patanjali's Sutra 2.35 (opposite page), that if we recognize and let go feelings of anger, hatred, resentment within ourselves, then we do not need to turn them back on others, so that forgiveness of ourselves will radiate out to those around us. Is not this what Nelson Mandela put into practice so brilliantly when he became President of South Africa? Experiments have been carried out, such as in Brighton, in the South of England, when there was violence coming into the town from people on motorbikes, a group meditated on a vision of the town restored to some peace; and the violence ceased. When they stopped the group meditation for a while, the violence returned and then stopped again when it resumed!

However it might be our path to be physically there doing something about the injustices in the world, or sitting in this way of contemplation might enable us to take on such a brave course of action as 'sitting' is a brave course of action in itself. This needs to be remembered when we undertake

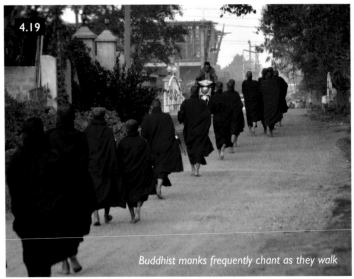

4.19

Buddhist monks frequently chant as they walk

what is a lifetime's path: an awareness, a consciousness of how we are.

Nirvana, a word that has been bandied about in the last few years, even as the name of a pop group, literally means 'to unbind'. The Buddha used many common everyday Pali words to best give a grasp of his meanings. I use this word, unbind, regularly when I am sitting. It can release an outer holding on, in the surface musculature of the body and touch me into the deep heart essence of being then taken out to a feeling of 'unbounded consciousness'.

There is a chant which encompasses this word. It is very profound, and gives the very core of why we would do the practices given throughout the book for the sake of the whole of humanity. The words of it are:

From the goodness that arises from my practice,
may my spiritual teachers and guides of great virtue,
my mother and my father and my relatives,
the sun and the moon and all virtuous leaders of the world,
the highest gods and evil forces, celestial beings,
guardian spirits of the earth, and the lord of death;
may those who are friendly, indifferent or hostile receive the blessing of my life, attain the
threefold bliss and realize the deathless.
From the goodness that arises from my practice and through this act of sharing may all desires
and attachments quickly cease and all harmful states of mind, until I reach nirvana.
In every kind of life may I have an upright mind, with mindfulness and vigour.
May darkness and delusion be dispelled.

THE CHANTING BOOK OF CHITHURST THERAVADA BUDDHIST MONASTERY

Chanting has long been a way to focus and still the mind in many spiritual practices and religions – the Sanskrit language has a special resonance to it that aligns the nadis (energy lines rather like a magnet field or acupuncture meridians).

When you chant, it is helpful to begin by sounding a clear sound with your mouth wide open – *Ahhhh*. On the same breath, let your lips come in but keep the openness of your mouth, so the sounds naturally becomes *Uhhh*. Then, let your lips lightly close so the sound becomes *Mmmmm*.

Stay with this sound A-U-M, repeating it until it naturally becomes *Om*. If you wish you can then bring in a whole Sanskrit chant, such as the *gayatri* mantra, the words of which are:

Om   Bhur   Bhuvah   Suvah
Tat   Savitur   Varenyam
Bhargo   Devasya   Dhimahi
Dhiyo   yo   Nah   Pracodayat

This chant acknowledges the rising of the sun for a new day and the setting of the sun to end the day and the Source that is behind that movement and the Universe. These times are traditionally considered auspicious times to meditate as there is a clear energy then. It has been translated in this way:

Let us contemplate the radiant Source of all Light:
may our minds merge with It,
thereby awakening our perception and understanding
on all three planes – physical, vital and mental.

(RIG VEDA **3-62-10**; YAJUR VEDA **3-63**)

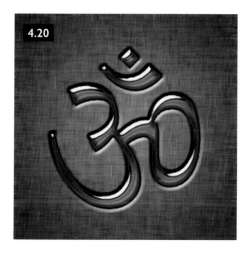

4.20

Books Mentioned or Recommended

THE ANATOMY OF MOVEMENT: Blandine Calais-Germain. Princeton, NJ, 2008

AWAKENING THE SPINE: Vanda Scaravelli. Pinter and Martin, London, 2011

BETWEEN EXTREMES: Brian Keenan and John Mccarthy. Black Swan, London, 2000

THE BHAGAVAD GITA translated by Swami Prabhavanda and Christopher Isherwood. Vedanta Press, London, 1956

THE BREATHING BOOK: Donna Farhi. Holt, USA, 1996

THE CHANTING BOOK: Chithurst Buddhist Monastery. Amaravati, Sussex, 1987

THE CONCISE BOOK OF MUSCLES: Chris Jarmey. Lotus Publishing, 2015

DON'T HOLD YOUR BREATH: Jenny Beeken. Polair, London, 2004

THE EMOTION CODE: Dr Bradley Nelson. Wellness Unmasked Publishing, 2007

THE GRASMERE JOURNALS: Dorothy Wordsworth. World's Classics, Oxford, 2007

I MET A MONK: Rose Elliot. Watkins, London, 2015

LIKE A FLOWER: Sandra Sabatini. Pinter and Martin, London, 2011

PERSON-CENTRED PSYCHOTHERAPIES: David J. Cain. American Psychological Association, 2010

THE SPECTRUM OF CONSCIOUSNESS: Ken Wilber. Quest Books, USA, 1996

THE THINKING BODY: Mabel Elsworth Todd. Dance Horizons, 1978

THE WILD PLACES: Robert Macfarlane. Granta Books, 2008

THE YOGA SUTRAS OF PATANJALI, translated by Alistair Shearer. Rider, London, 2010

VIPASSANA MEDITATION: see www.dhamma.org

[continued from p. 80] IYT Teacher, I offer yoga classes for children from the age of four to elderly 'Evergreens', now in their nineties.

My thanks to John for giving me the space and patience during this period of time as I worked on these drawings, under Jenny's guidance. The illustrations have come from an inner knowledge and heartfelt awareness of the Inner Yoga Trust teachings.

Models in the Posture Pictures

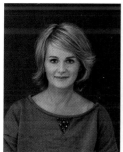 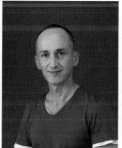 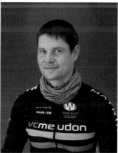 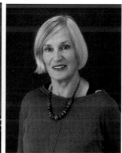 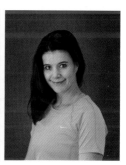

| *Lisa Christensen* | *Thierry Lambert* | *Will Lane* | *Jenny Beeken* | *Patricia Lopez* |

Photo credits

All photographs illustrating posture except those on pp. 32-4, plus those on this page, are by Michael Prior Studio
Photographs p. 9 by Jane Stockton; Contracted six-pack, p. 24: Wikimedia Commons/Berni1992
Cycling and climbing pictures: of Will Lane (p. 32) by Michael Prior; of Robert Barnes (p. 33) by Le Domestic Tours and of Adam Brickley (p. 34) by Christina Thiele
Seated Statue of Pharaoh's Daughter Nefret-iabet, 4th Dynasty, p. 58: Wikimedia Commons/Captmondo;
Skeleton, p. 65: Science Photo Library; Spectrum of visible light, p. 66: Wikimedia Commons;
Monks chanting, p. 76, by Rob Hodgson; Red rose, p. 68: Laitche [CC BY-SA 4.0 (http://creativecommons.org/licenses/by-sa/4.0) or FAL], via Wikimedia Commons; Buddha, p. 75: mygodpictures.com; Golden aum, p. 76: Wikimedia Commons; Jenny Beeken, p. 80: James Beeken

About the Contributors

Jenny Beeken (author):

I first woke up to an awareness of my body when I went on intensive courses in Pune, India with Shri B. K. S. Iyengar in 1979 and 1981. Since then I have had a regular daily practice to maintain and increase that awareness together with awareness of how I stand, walk and sit in my day-to-day life. This makes me very aware of how we all tend to hold ourselves.

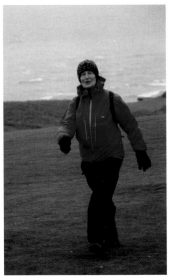

I have been teaching yoga, awareness and meditation since 1979, and have become increasingly aware of how we can transform our posture, breathing and mind and so our health through a daily practice and an awareness of how we live our life.

As I completed this book, I went on a six-day walk along the South Downs Way, from where I live in Hampshire to Beachy Head – to put all that is contained here into my walking.

Patricia (Pachi) Lopez (co-author):

I took up yoga and running seriously almost at the same time and I have been practising both since then. It was around six years ago that I decided to become a yoga teacher with the Inner Yoga Trust. Since then I have been mainly teaching yoga to athletes.

I became a Coach in Running Fitness with the UKA and ran two road marathons, an off-road marathon and the Snowdon Trail Marathon, which was an ultramarathon, among many other races. I also became a vipassana meditator. My running coaching comes from within, where yoga and meditation are the biggest part of it. For me yoga and running go alongside: they complement each other and they fulfil my life.

Murray Ana Nettle (illustrator):

I trained as a figurative artist, and went on to take my Bachelor of Art in Fine Art Sculpture at the Central School of Art in London (now part of the University of the Arts).

I live with my husband John and Milly our Jack Russell terrier in the village of Harting under the South Downs. I first practised yoga in 1989 under Jenny Beeken's guidance, when pregnant with the third of my four children, and since then have been taught solely by Jenny and other core Inner Yoga Trust tutors. Having now acquired my own qualification as an [to p. 79]